the best of the

APPALACHIAN

trail   *OVERNIGHT*

HIKES

Book list

Also by Victoria and Frank Logue

THE BEST OF THE APPALACHIAN TRAIL: OVERNIGHT HIKES

THE APPALACHIAN TRAIL HIKER

APPALACHIAN TRAIL FUN BOOK

Also by Victoria Logue

HIKING AND BACKPACKING: ESSENTIAL SKILLS TO ADVANCED TECHNIQUES

GUIDE TO THE BLUE RIDGE PARKWAY

Also by Leonard M. Adkins

THE APPALACHIAN TRAIL: A VISITOR'S COMPANION

WILDFLOWERS OF THE APPALACHIAN TRAIL

WALKING THE BLUE RIDGE:
A GUIDE TO THE TRAILS OF THE BLUE RIDGE PARKWAY

50 HIKES IN SOUTHERN VIRGINIA:
FROM THE CUMBERLAND GAP TO THE ATLANTIC OCEAN

50 HIKES IN NORTHERN VIRGINIA: WALKS, HIKES, AND BACKPACKS
FROM THE ALLEGHENY MOUNTAINS TO THE CHESAPEAKE BAY

50 HIKES IN MARYLAND: WALKS, HIKES, AND BACKPACKS FROM THE
ALLEGHENY PLATEAU TO THE ATLANTIC OCEAN

MARYLAND: AN EXPLORER'S GUIDE

ADVENTURE GUIDE TO VIRGINIA

THE CARIBBEAN: A WALKING AND HIKING GUIDE

WILDFLOWERS OF THE BLUE RIDGE AND GREAT SMOKY MOUNTAINS

the best of the

APPALACHIAN

trail *OVERNIGHT*

HIKES

SECOND EDITION

Victoria and Frank Logue with
Leonard M. Adkins

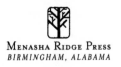

MENASHA RIDGE PRESS
BIRMINGHAM, ALABAMA

APPALACHIAN TRAIL CONSERVANCY
HARPERS FERRY, WEST VIRGINIA

The hikes in this book describe the route of the Appalachian Trail at the time of publication. The Trail is occasionally relocated and the route may differ at the time of your hike. Severe damage to the Trail caused by storms may impact your hike as well. If the white blazes differ from the hike described in this book, follow the Trail as it is marked. Neither the authors nor the publishers can guarantee your safety on the hikes described in this book. Use caution and your best judgment.

NOTE: Water sources are identified for hikers' convenience, but this is not an endorsement of their purity. All water should be treated before consuming.

Copyright © 1994, 2004 by Victoria and Frank Logue and Leonard M. Adkins

All rights reserved

Printed in Canada

Published by Menasha Ridge Press and The Appalachian Trail Conservancy

Distributed by Publishers Group West

Second edition, second printing, 2008

Cover photo by GOODSHOOT/Alamy

Text and design by Palace Press International

Cartography by Travis Bryant

Typesetting by Annie Long

Library of Congress Cataloging-in-Publication Data
Logue, Victoria, 1961–

The best of the Appalachian trail : overnight hikes / Victoria and Frank Logue with Leonard Adkins.—2nd ed.

p.cm.

ISBN 10: 0-89732-528-1

ISBN 13: 978-0-89732-528-8

1. Hiking—Appalachian Trail—Guidebooks. 2. Backpacking—Appalachian Trail—Guidebooks.
3. Appalachian Trail—Guidebooks. I. Logue, Frank, 1963– II. Adkins, Leonard M. III. Title.

GV199.42.A68L65 2004

796.51'0974--dc22   20040948042

Menasha Ridge Press

P.O. Box 43673

Birmingham, AL 35243

www.menasharidge.com

Appalachian Trail Conservancy

P.O. Box 807

Harpers Ferry, WV 25425

www.appalachiantrail.org

For my mother, Nancy Adkins:
her strength and determination put A.T. thru-hikers to shame.—Leonard

For Willie Frank Logue, the best grandmother a boy could have.—Frank

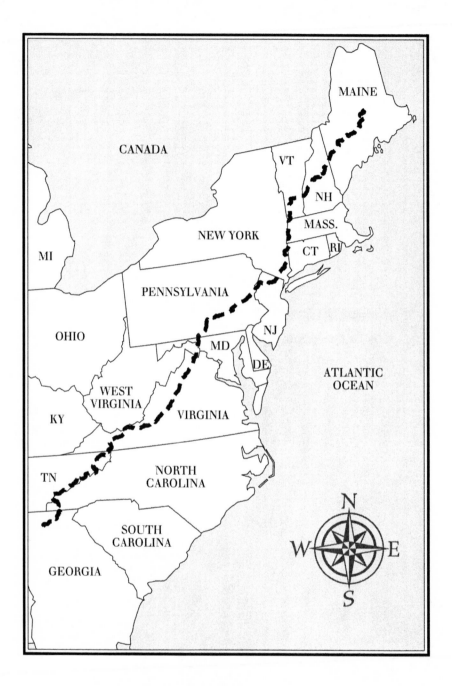

THE APPALACHIAN TRAIL

CONTENTS

ACKNOWLEDGMENTS

A BOOK IS NEVER THE WORK OF THE AUTHOR OR AUTHORS ALONE. WE WISH TO .ACKNOWLEDGE AND THANK THE MANY PEOPLE WHO TOOK TIME OUT OF THEIR BUSY SCHEDULES TO ASSIST US.

FRANK AND VICTORIA GIVE THEIR HEARTFELT THANKS TO LEONARD FOR TAKING ON THE LION'S SHARE OF THIS PROJECT, WHICH MADE KEEPING THESE BOOKS UP-TO-DATE POSSIBLE.

LEONARD WOULD LIKE TO THANK: MICHAEL ALPER, BATONA HIKING CLUB; NANCY D. ANTHONY, NATURAL BRIDGE APPALACHIAN TRAIL CLUB; JEFF BUEHLER, SUSQUEHANNA APPALACHIAN TRAIL CLUB; V. COLLINS CHEW, TENNESSEE EASTMAN HIKING CLUB; KITTY FARLEY, MOUNT ROGERS APPALACHIAN TRAIL CLUB; DORIS GOVE, SMOKY MOUNTAINS HIKING CLUB; EDWARD F. KENNA, JR., PHILADELPHIA TRAIL CLUB; HOWARD MCDONALD, CAROLINA MOUNTAIN CLUB; ANDREW NORKIN, AMC WHITE MOUNTAINS TRAILS MANAGER; HERBERT OGDEN, GREEN MOUNTAIN CLUB; CHARLES PERRY, ROANOKE APPALACHIAN TRAIL CLUB; BILL ROGERS, TIDEWATER APPALACHIAN TRAIL CLUB; LEE SHEAFFER, POTOMAC APPALACHIAN TRAIL CLUB; VAUGHN THOMAS, PIEDMONT APPALACHIAN TRAIL HIKERS; MELANIE WERTZ, CUMBERLAND VALLEY APPALACHIAN TRAIL MANAGEMENT ASSOCIATION— THANK YOU FOR CHECKING THE MANUSCRIPTS FOR ACCURACY. ANY ERRORS THAT MAY REMAIN ARE OURS AND NOT YOURS.

BRIAN B. KING, ATC DIRECTOR OF PUBLIC AFFAIRS—THANKS FOR YOUR SUPPORT THROUGH THE MANY YEARS.

DR. STEPHEN LEWIS, CAROLINE CHARONKO, TERRY CUMMING, AND SUSIE SURFAS—THANK YOU FOR THE MANY EXTRA YEARS OF TRAIL LIFE YOU HAVE GIVEN ME.

NANCY ADKINS—LOVE YOU FOREVER, MOM.

KATHLEEN, JOHN, TIM, AND JAY YELENIC—LOVE YOU TOO.

LAURIE—WHO COULD EVER HAVE IMAGINED I WOULD FIND YOU? YOU ARE MY PERFECT COMPANION THROUGH THE TRAILS OF LIFE.

INTRODUCTION

DAWN IS STRETCHING HER ROSY LIMBS, SLENDER PINK FINGERS CARESSING THE GRASSY PLAIN AROUND OUR TENT. THE SURREAL NIGHT—VELVET-BLACK SKY WITH CRESCENT MOON, FERAL PONIES GRAZING, THE INSISTENT DRIP OF DEW—FADES AS DAYLIGHT ILLUMINATES THE SLEEPING WORLD. EXCEPT FOR THE PONIES, WE ARE ALONE.

WILBURN RIDGE NEAR GRAYSON HIGHLANDS IN VIRGINIA IS AN EXQUISITELY BEAUTIFUL AREA TO CAMP. YOU MUST BACKPACK TO GET THERE AND IT IS WORTH EVERY STRAINING MUSCLE TO ASCEND THE RIDGE. GRASSY MEADOWS, CLUMPS OF FIR, ROCK OUTCROPPINGS AND WILD PONIES DECORATE THE TABLEAU BEFORE YOU, NOT UNLIKE A MONET LANDSCAPE.

IMPRESSIONISM, SURREALISM AND REALISM COMBINED, THE HIGHLANDS ARE ALWAYS READY FOR AN ARTIST'S BRUSH. FROM THE GREAT STORMS THAT CRASH AND ROAR OVER MOUNT ROGERS TO THE WEST TO THE PALETTE OF COLORS THAT PAINT THE LANDSCAPE AS THE SUN RISES IN THE EAST, YOU CANNOT TAKE THIS PLACE FOR GRANTED. AS YOU HIKE THE APPALACHIAN TRAIL (A.T.) ACROSS GRAYSON HIGHLANDS AND OVER WILBURN RIDGE TO RHODODENDRON GAP, THE PANORAMA IS AWE INSPIRING. MORE THAN TWO MILES FROM WHERE WE SET UP CAMP, WE COULD STILL SEE THE TENT'S SILHOUETTE ON THE RIDGE, THE WILD PONIES NOSING AND TASTING THE ALIEN STRUCTURE.

OUR DAUGHTER, GRIFFIN, ENJOYED THE PONIES, IMITATING THE HEEL-KICKING FOALS THAT WHICKERED AND NEIGHED AS THEY CHASED EACH OTHER ABOUT THE MEADOW. SHE PICKED DAISIES, EXPLORED ROCK GROUPINGS, AND FINALLY SETTLED DOWN SNUG IN HER SLEEPING BAG AS DUSK BLANKETED THE MEADOWS.

THIS IS JUST ONE OF MANY EXPERIENCES POSSIBLE WHEN HIKING OVERNIGHT ALONG THE A.T., EXPERIENCES WE HOPE THIS BOOK WILL HELP YOU ENCOUNTER.

History of the Appalachian Trail

The idea for a trail running the length of the Appalachian Mountains was first considered in the twentieth century. The Appalachian Trail, as we know it, was the vision of Benton MacKaye (rhymes with sky) and others who had been thinking about the concept for more than ten years. In 1921, MacKaye took the initiative and launched the project through an article in *The Journal of the American Institute of Architects.*

MacKaye wrote about the purpose of the Trail: "There would be a chance to catch a breath, to study the dynamic forces of nature and the possibilities of shifting to them the burdens now carried on the backs of men . . . Industry would come to be seen in its true perspective as a means in life and not as an end in itself."

MacKaye's original intent was to construct a trail from "the highest peak in the North to the highest peak in the South-from Mount Washington (New Hampshire) to Mount Mitchell (North Carolina)." He envisioned a fourfold plan including the trail, shelters, community camps, and food and farm camps. The camps never came about. And although MacKaye's larger economic plan for the Appalachian Trail never gained support, his main purpose-an opportunity for American families to commune with nature-is the reason for the Trail's continuing existence today.

Within a year after MacKaye's article appeared in the architectural journal, the New York-New Jersey Trail Conference began work on a new trail with the goal of making it part of the Appalachian Trail. In the Hudson River Valley, the new Bear Mountain Bridge would connect the future section in New England with Harriman State Park and eventually with Delaware Water Gap in Pennsylvania.

In 1925, MacKaye and others formed the Appalachian Trail Conference (ATC) to guide the project to completion. By 1936, Myron H. Avery, who would be president of the Appalachian Trail Conference for 20 years, had finished measuring the flagged route of the Appalachian Trail. He became the first 2,000-miler a year before the completion of the Trail.

On August 14, 1937, the Civilian Conservation Corps (CCC) workers cleared the final link in the 2,025-mile Appalachian Trail. On a high ridge connecting Spaulding and Sugarloaf Mountains in Maine, a six-person CCC crew cut the last two miles of trail. The finished route of the Appalachian Trail was not as originally envisioned by MacKaye; the final product was longer, stretching from Mount Oglethorpe (the southern terminus of the eastern Blue Ridge) in Georgia to Katahdin in Maine's Baxter State Park.

The trail did not remain complete for long. The next year, a hurricane demolished miles of trail in the northeast, while the decision to connect the Skyline Drive (under construction at the time) with the Blue Ridge Parkway displaced another 120 miles of trail in Virginia. The trail was not made continuous again until 1951, after the world had settled down from World War II.

In 1968, President Lyndon Johnson signed the National Trails System Act and made the Appalachian Trail the first National Scenic Trail. The act charged federal agencies with the task of buying lands to protect the trailway from encroaching development, but ten years passed before the government acted and began protecting the trail lands. At the beginning of 2004, only 10.7 miles of the A.T. remained to be protected.

Perhaps the most amazing aspect of the world's largest greenway is that the

Trail was conceived and developed by private citizens. As a testament to the work carried out for decades by volunteers, the federal government left the management of the Trail to a private nonprofit group—the Appalachian Trail Conference—even after the footpath was brought under federal protection.

SELECTING A HIKE

The A.T. now offers more than 2,100 miles of hiking possibilities, from scenic rambles along rivers to strenuous scrambles up rocky peaks. The descriptions of hikes in this book often suggest more than great hikes.

The information provided will also tell you good times to hike in the area or when to avoid hiking there. Interesting flora and fauna is mentioned as is notable history. To help you pick out a hike that offers just what you are looking for, several easy-to-find pieces of information are located at the top of each hike description: the hike rating, length and time of the hike, and icons denoting major attractions along the way.

ICONS

Each hike has one or more icons that show the major attractions along the way. The icons (mountain peak, scenic view, pond or river, waterfall, historic area, or bird-watching area) are intended to give you an easy-to-identify symbol that you can use when you flip through the book looking for a hike.

MOUNTAIN PEAK

SCENIC VIEW

POND OR RIVER

WHEELCHAIR ACCESSIBLE

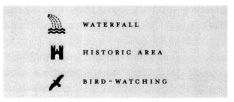

WATERFALL

HISTORIC AREA

BIRD-WATCHING

RATINGS

The hikes are rated as easy, moderate, or strenuous. Easy denotes hikes with little elevation gain or loss that are not more than ten miles in length. Moderate hikes have no long, steep climbs or descents but there may be some short, steep grades or long, gradual ascents. Strenuous hikes are steep, and sometimes long, and should not be attempted by inexperienced hikers or people in poor physical condition.

HIKE LENGTH

To gauge hiking time on the trail, allow a half-hour for each mile as well as an additional hour for each thousand feet of elevation gain. This pace allows for a leisurely hike with some time to stop at points of interest. The hikes can certainly be done faster or slower, but this formula will give you an idea of the time you'll need.

Many of these hikes are traverses, beginning at one point and ending at a second. All traverses require that you be shuttled or that you have someone drop you off and pick you up.

EQUIPMENT FOR OVERNIGHT HIKES

To go on an overnight backpacking trip, there are several pieces of equipment that you need beyond what you carry on a day hike. The plethora of equipment out there may seem daunting at first, but basically all you need is food, water, and shelter. Many backpacking stores have equipment available for rent so that you can try the gear, and sport, out before you invest in new equipment. For a good book on the subject, try Victoria Logue's *Backpacking: Essential Skills to Advanced Techniques*. Available from most outdoor retailers and many bookstores, it covers the latest equipment as well as time-honored skills for backcountry travel. 🖎

Boots

Hiking boots range in price from $50 to $250 and are generally divided into three categories: heavyweight, mediumweight, and lightweight. Heavyweight boots, which weigh more than four pounds, are generally designed for technically demanding climbs on ice (usually with crampons) or on snow or alpine rock. You will not need heavyweights for the hikes in this book unless you choose to climb Katahdin in the dead of winter.

Mediumweight boots, which weigh from 2.5 to 4 pounds, are almost entirely made of leather, though many blend in a combination of tough fabric as well. Mediumweights are ideal for the broadest range of hiking situations.

Lightweight boots, which weigh less than 2.5 pounds, are almost always made with a combination of leather and a "breathable" fabric. Lightweights rarely require a "breaking-in" period and are tough enough to handle any of the hikes in this book.

When purchasing a boot, the important factor to keep in mind is proper fit. Even the best boots will make you miserable if they are not fitted properly. This is best done in a store, but you can also purchase boots by mail order if the company has a good return policy. Once you buy the boots, make sure to break them in well around town before heading out into the woods. If lightweights fit properly, they won't require a breaking in, but even these boots can be purchased too small or too big, too narrow or too wide. Be prepared with moleskin to treat "hot spots" before blisters develop. 🖎

Backpacks

Backpacks cost between $50 and $400 and are divided into two categories: internal frame and external frame. The external frame pack is designed to distribute weight equally with a high center of gravity, perfect for established trails. An external pack is cooler to wear because it rides away from your back. The internal frame pack is designed to custom-fit the hiker and has a low center of gravity, which makes it popular for off-trail hiking and mountaineering.

An important feature when purchasing a pack is the hip belt. Since the hip belt will carry most of the pack's weight, it should be well padded. Also make sure that it is well built and snug-fitting. 🖎

Sleeping Bags

Because you will spend one third of your time in a sleeping bag when backpacking, it is important to get a good one. The factors to consider include: comfort rating, filling, weight, and shape. The comfort rating provided by the manufacturer gives the lowest temperature at which the bag will still be comfortable. The filling may be goose down or a synthetic, such as Hollofil, PolarGuard HV, or Lite Loft. Down gives the most warmth for the weight of the bag, but synthetics provide more warmth when wet. Mummy-shaped bags are the most popular with backpackers because they offer the most warmth and space for the weight. Rectangular bags offer more space but weigh more and provide less warmth than mummy bags. Good sleeping bags range in price from $75 to $400. 🖎

Tents

A tent provides protection from bugs and the elements, and is an important purchase. Features to take into consideration include: weight, room, ventilation, and "ease-of-setup." For backpacking, you will not want to carry more than four pounds of tent per person.

When looking at tent size, you will need to decide whether you want to hang your gear up outside the tent or keep it in the tent with you. A two-person tent has room for two people, and if you want to bring your gear inside, you'll need a three-person tent. If you intend to do a lot of summer hiking, a well-ventilated tent is an absolute necessity. Most tents today offer plenty of no-see-um netting for cross ventilation and protection from bugs. Make sure the tent you purchase is well-ventilated.

How easily you can set your tent up and take it back down is another important consideration. Practice helps, but if your tent is difficult to set up, you may end up getting soaked in a sudden storm. Good backpacking tents (two or three-person) range in price from $100 to $400.

Equipment Checklist

- Hiking boots
- Backpack
- Sleeping bag
- Sleeping pad
- Tent/tarp, and ground cloth
- Stove and fuel
- Cooking pot and eating utensils
- Pocket knife
- Water filter or iodine (unless you plan to boil your water)
- Food for length of hike
- Spices*
- One-liter (minimum) water bottle
- Drinking cup
- Fluorescent/blaze orange clothing, vest, hat , or pack cover
- Raingear and pack cover
- Gaiters*
- One pair of shorts
- One pair of loose-fitting long pants*
- One or two short-sleeved shirts
- One long-sleeved shirt or sweater
- Knit cap
- Balaclava
- Down or synthetic fill parka*
- Two pairs of liner socks
- Two pairs of hiking socks
- Bandannas
- Long johns*
- Two pair of underwear*
- Toilet paper and trowel
- Biodegradable soap and washcloth
- Deodorant*
- Toothbrush and toothpaste
- Shaving kit*
- Nylon cord (at least 50 feet)
- Maps and guidebooks
- Compass
- Flashlight with new batteries
- Watch or clock*
- Sunglasses*
- First-aid kit (including moleskin and space blanket)
- Emergency phone numbers
- Copy of itinerary (original left at home with family members)
- Swimsuit and towel*
- Extra shoes*
- Repair supplies for pack, tent, and stove*
- Camera and film*
- Radio with headphones*
- Insect repellent
- Sunscreen and lotion*
- Hiking stick*
- Crampons and ice axe*

Additional Equipment for Longer Hikes

- Repair equipment for clothes
- Trash bag

An extra long-sleeved shirt or sweater
Long johns
Reading material*
Journal*

optional or seasonal equipment

Minimum Impact

Minimum impact camping is a philosophy once summed up by the National Park Service as, "Take nothing but pictures, leave nothing but footprints." The following sub-headings discuss measures to help eliminate traces of your presence along the Trail. This is not a list of rules but rather a way of living that is becoming increasingly important to adopt. If these techniques are not used by everyone (and currently they're not), the A.T. will lose its natural beauty. Nature is resilient, but its ability to fight back is limited. A little bit of help goes a long way toward improving the world we're escaping to. If everyone pitches in, we'll be able to enjoy our backcountry experiences even more.

Carry Out All of Your Trash

Pack it in, pack it out, and you're already one giant step toward keeping the environment clean. Store your trash in a sack. Trash includes everything, even organic material. Orange peels, apple cores and eggshells may strike you as natural trash, easily biodegradable. Why not toss it into the brush? Because it takes five months for an orange peel to rot and become one with the earth.

There is nothing worse than heading into the woods to relieve yourself and discovering a trail of paper proving you weren't the first at this spot. Soggy, used toilet paper is probably one of the uglier reminders of human presence.

Following trails littered with cigarette butts is disheartening. If you want to smoke, that's your prerogative, but don't think of the outdoors as one big ashtray. Not only is the litter of cigarette butts ugly, but it only takes one stray spark to start a forest fire that will turn the woods into a huge ashtray.

Carry Out Trash Left by Others

For some reason, people who wouldn't dare throw trash on the ground at home do so freely in the outdoors. Unfortunately, the enviro-conscious do not outnumber the users and abusers of America's trails. We have to make up for their ignorance and sloth by picking up after them.

You can make the outdoors a better place by stopping occasionally to pick up other people's trash. You don't have to be ridiculous and carry out nasty toilet paper or rotting organic material, but take a minute to cover it with leaves, moss, dirt, and twigs. Pick up trash, you'll find you feel a lot better about yourself.

Switchbacks

Stay on designated trails; switchbacks are there for a reason. They slow down the Trail erosion on steep climbs. It may seem easier to scramble up the hillside to the next section of trail, but if too many people did that, waterways would use the newly exposed earth as a water course washing away both trail and mountain in its wake. You may curse the person who blazed it and those who attempt to keep it passable for you, but remember that just about any trail you hike was built and maintained by volunteers.

Solid-Waste Management

In other words, how to dispose of your excrement. Disposing of your feces when backpacking is absolutely necessary. Always, always, always (I can't say it too many times) dig a hole. More importantly, make sure you're at least 200 feet from the nearest water source. If you're hiking alongside a stream, climb up. There's more to being green than just packing out your trash. Disposing properly of your solid waste will keep the wilderness much more appealing. ❧

TRAIL MAINTENANCE

Give back to the Trail and the hiking community by becoming involved in trail maintenance. Maintaining a section of existing trail or helping out with blazing new trails is a good way to pay back the outdoors for the good times you have received from it. Trails are beginning to crisscross the entire country, and there is sure to be a new or old trail somewhere near you. Contact your local trail clubs to see what you can do to help out. Most backpacking shops can tell you about clubs in your area.

The Appalachian Trail is maintained by volunteers. Contact the Appalachian Trail Conservancy or ATC (see Appendix) to find out more about helping maintain the Appalachian Trail. ❧

FINDING SOLITUDE

Many hikers retreat to the Appalachian Trail seeking a wilderness experience, only to find themselves on a crowded section of trail sharing their "wilderness experience" with more hikers than they bargained for. Here are a few tips for finding a little solitude on America's most popular long distance trail.

Start your hike early in the morningor on days that are not during the peak time. There is something about being alone on a summit—just you and a a spectacular view. That was on a Labor Day weekend, when later in the day hikers marched in a long, single-file line from Baxter Peak to Parnola Peak. By making an effort to get up early (and hike the tricky section of trail in the dark), we had the peak to ourselves on perhaps the busiest day of the year.

Another way to find your own piece of the Appalachian Trail is to hike during the off-season. Roan Highlands on the Tennessee–North Carolina state line is very crowded during peak bloom of the rhododendron garden.

In June, visitors flock to see the awesome spectacle-thousands of big catawba rhododendrons in bloom at once-but during the winter we have camped alone on the summit. We didn't see the rhododendrons in bloom, but the snow-covered mountain was a magnificent sight.

A third way to find solitude on the country's most popular long distance trail is to discover your own special places. After enjoying the hikes in this book, branch out and discover more of the Trail on your own. To help you in your search, the Appalachian Trail Conservancy publishes a set of eleven guidebooks. They cover the entire 2,100-mile footpath, mile by mile. ❧

SAFETY

Trouble is rare on the Appalachian Trail, but theft is not uncommon. Cars parked at trailheads are usually targeted for break-ins because thieves know that the owner will be away for awhile, Do not leave visible anything worth stealing, or better yet, leave all valuables at home. Also, do not leave any notes on your car stating where you are going and how long you intend to be gone. You might as well advertise for your car to be broken into.

It is doubtful you will run into any troublesome humans on the A.T., but if you do run into someone that gives you a bad feeling, keep moving. Weather is something else you need to be concerned about when hiking. While it is neither impossible nor necessarily uncomfortable to hike in rain or snow or intense heat, there are certain precautions you should take. Clothing suitable to the situation is important-raingear for rain, layered clothing for snow and cold weather, and lightweight, porous clothing for hot days. With the appropriate clothing, you can go a long ways toward avoiding both hypothermia and hyperthermia.

Some of the hikes mentioned in this book are along sections of trail that are above tree line or in other exposed areas. In some cases, an alternate bad weather route is available, but in many places, this is not an option. If inclement weather is predicted, it might be wise to take a rain check. For above tree line hikes, carry along raingear just in case because storms can form suddenly at high elevations.

Getting lost is rarely a problem on the A.T., but anyone can become distracted and miss a blaze that indicates a turn. The Appalachian Trail is marked with white blazes at least every quarter mile, and usually more often. Most maintainers try to blaze so you can see the next blaze as soon as you have passed the previous one. So, if you have walked for more than five minutes without seeing a blaze, it would be wise to backtrack until you see a blaze and then continue on your way.

First Aid
The risk of serious injury on a day hike is not high, but being unprepared would be tempting fate. You can still get stung by a bee, twist an ankle, develop blisters, become hypothermic or have a heat stroke. The following information will give you some ideas about how to deal with these situations if they arise.

Hypothermia
Shivering, numbness, drowsiness and marked muscular weakness are the first signs of hypothermia. These symptoms are followed by mental confusion, impairment of judgement, slurred speech, failing eyesight and unconsciousness. The most serious warning sign of hypothermia occurs when the shivering stops. If the victim stops shivering, he is close to death.

Fortunately, hypothermia is easy to treat. If you or a friend is feeling hypothermic, get warm. In the case of a day hike, this may mean nothing more than hurrying back to your car, stripping yourself of wet clothes, and turning the heater on. If you are hiking with friends, they may be able to help you get warm. As long as you are hiking, your body will continue to try and warm itself. Keeping still could mean death, unless you are taking action to warm back up.

Hyperthermia
This ailment develops in three steps: heat cramps, heat exhaustion and heat stroke. The best treatment for hyperthermia is prevention. If you are hiking in particularly hot weather, make sure you maintain a continual and consistent intake of fluids. Dehydration is what usually leads to heat-related ailments. Also, if hiking is making you too hot, take a break, find some shade, drink some water, and give your body a few minutes to cool off.

If you progress to heat cramps (legs or abdomen begin to cramp), you are on your way to heat exhaustion and heat stroke. Take a break and sip water slowly. It is best to add a bit of salt to the water if possible. Rather than continue hiking, you should call it a day, and if possible, return to your car.

Heat exhaustion can follow heat cramps. Although the body temperature remains fairly normal, the skin is pale, cool, and clammy; you may also feel faint, weak, nauseated, and dizzy. Sit in the shade and sip water. Lower your head between your knees to relieve the dizziness. You can also lie down, loosen or take off your clothes, and elevate your feet about one foot. Bathe in cool water if there if possible. Vomiting signals a serious condition and medical help should be sought.

When suffering from heat stroke, the skin becomes hot, red and dry; the pulse, rapid and strong. Unconsciousness is common. The victim should be undressed and bathed in cool water until the skin temperature is lowered, but do not over chill the victim, which can be as dangerous as overheating. Medical attention should be sought as soon as possible.

Blisters

Blisters develop slowly and can make you miserable. As soon as you feel a hot spot, cover it with moleskin. If not treated properly, blisters can become infected. If you do get a blister, leave it unbroken; if it is already broken, treat it like an open wound, cleansing it and bandaging it. Do not continue to hike if you are in too much pain.

Lightning

Lightning kills more people each year than any other natural disaster, including earthquakes, floods and tornadoes. If you get caught on the Trail during a lightning storm, there are a few things you can do to reduce your chances of being struck. Avoid bodies of water and low places where water can collect. Avoid high places, ridges, open places, tall objects, metal objects, rock outcroppings, wet caves and ditches. If possible, find a stand of trees and sit with your knees pulled up to your chest, head bowed and arms hugging knees.

Bee Stings

Although most insects (other than black flies, deer flies, and ticks) will try to avoid you, bees (yellow jackets in particular) are attracted to food, beverages, perfume, scented soaps and lotions, deodorant, and bright-colored (and dark) clothing. Yellow jackets nest anywhere that provides cover-logs, trees, even underground And they don't mind stinging more than once!

If you're sensitive to stings, carry an oral antihistamine to reduce swelling. A topical antihistamine, such as Benadryl, will help reduce itching. If you are allergic and a potential victim of anaphylactic, shock, carry an Anakit whenever you hike. The Anakit, which must be prescribed by a doctor, contains a couple of injections of epinephrine as well as antihistamine tablets. If you use the kit, seek medical attention as soon as possible.

Other Pests

Deer, bear, boar, moose, raccoons, snakes, skunk and porcupines can all be found along the A.T., but these animals rarely cause problems for hikers; particularly day hikers.

Bee stings, as discussed above, present an immediate and potentially fatal problem, but there are other insects on the Trail to watch out for no-see-ums, black flies, deer flies, horse flies, mosquitoes and ticks. The first five insects all produce itchy, painful bites that can be treated with a topical or oral antihistamine (or both, depending on how badly you react to their bites). Wearing lots of clothing, including a hat, will put the bugs at a disadvantage, but you may be comfortable. A bug repellent that is a 35 percent deet works best.

Along the A.T., the tick is the biggest problem because some are infected with Lyme disease. You will need to take a little extra precaution. The tiny (about the size of a pinhead) deer tick is the carrier of Lyme disease. Whenever you hike in tick country (tall grass and underderbrush), make sure you check yourself afterwards for ticks. It takes a while for a tick to become imbedded, so a thorough check at the end of the day will help you catch the tick before it catches you.

Wear a hat, long sleeve shirt, and pants with cuffs tucked into socks to discourage ticks. Too uncomfortable? Use a repellent with permethrin and stick to the center of the Trail to avoid brushing against branches and shrubs. Ticks, like mosquitoes, are attracted to heat and have been known to hang around for months waiting for a hot body to pass by. Try wearing light colored clothing so you'll be able to see the ticks more clearly.

If a tick attaches itself to your body, the best way to remove it is by grasping the skin directly below where the tick is attached and removing the tick along with a small piece of skin. Then carefully wash the bite with soap and water. Following its removal, keep an eye out for the symptoms of Lyme disease: fever, headache, and pain and stiffness in joints and muscles. If left untreated, Lyme disease can produce lifelong impairment of muscular and nervous systems, chronic arthritis, brain injury, and in 10 percent of victims, crippling arthritis. If you suspect Lyme, see your doctor. Tick season is from April to October with a peak from May to July.

HANTAVIRUS

This deadly disease made the news in 1994 with an outbreak in the Four Comers area of the southwest. About that time, the Trail community learned that an A.T. thru-hiker had contracted hantavirus about 18 months earlier while hiking through southwest Virginia. The hiker had been hospitalized for a month in 1992 with the disease, but returned to the A.T. in 1994 to complete his thru hike. Meanwhile, many hikers were left with grave concerns about this new infectious disease.

Hantavirus is rare and difficult to contract. You must have contact with the feces or urine of deer mice, or breathe air infected with the disease through evaporated droppings. Federal and state authorities have trapped and tested mice in shelters in southwest Virginia without finding evidence of the disease. To be safe, avoid all contact with mice and their droppings. Air out a closed, mice-infested structure an hour before occupying it.

DOGS

From the *Leave No Trace Southeast Skills and Ethics* booklet: *"Wildlife and pets are not a good mix—even on a leash, dogs harass wildlife and disturb other visitors . . . The best option is to leave dogs at home. Obedience champion or not, every dog is a potential carrier of diseases that infect wildlife."*

If you do take your dog, keep him on a leash to prevent him from chasing wildlife and dogs around other hikers. Dogs are required to be on a leash in many areas along the A.T.

THE APPALACHIAN TRAIL IN MAINE IS MORE RUGGED AND REMOTE THAN IN ANY OF THE OTHER 13 TRAIL STATES. THE NORTHERN TERMINUS OF THE A.T. IS AT BAXTER PEAK ON TOP OF KATAHDIN IN MAINE'S BAXTER STATE PARK. FROM THAT PEAK, YOU CAN LOOK TO THE SOUTHWEST AND SEE THE MAINE LAKE COUNTRY THAT THE A.T. CROSSES.

Maine

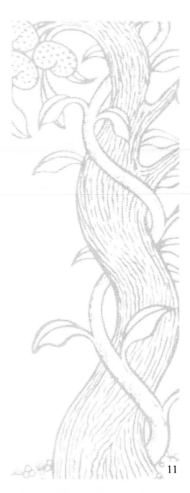

THE TRAIL IN MAINE TRAVERSES SEVERAL PROMINENT MOUNTAINS INCLUDING THE TWIN PEAKS OF THE BIGELOW RANGE, THE CROCKERS, SADDLEBACK, OLD BLUE, BALDPATES, AND THE MAHOOSUC RANGE. IN THE MAHOOSUCS, THE A.T. HAS WHAT IS OFTEN DESCRIBED AS THE "TOUGHEST MILE." THIS SECTION THROUGH MAHOOSUC NOTCH IS A TESTAMENT TO A TRAIL-BUILDER'S IMAGINATION AND A HIKER'S STAMINA; HERE THE A.T. GOES OVER AND UNDER INCREDIBLE-SIZED BOULDERS. THE A.T. CONTINUES OVER GOOSE EYE AND MOUNT CARLO ON ITS WAY TO THE STATE LINE OF NEW HAMPSHIRE.

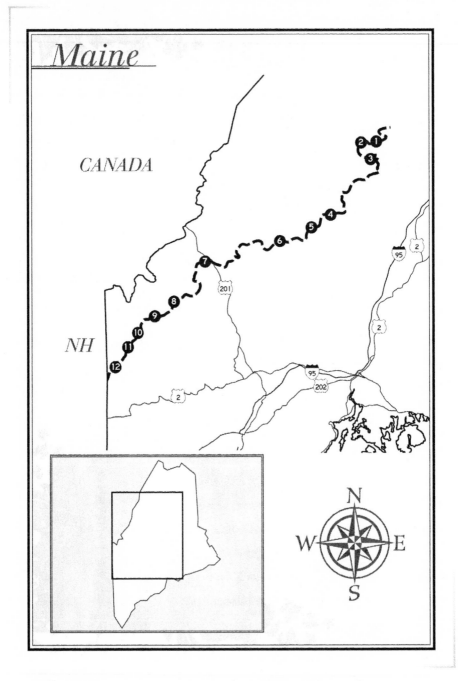

Maine

CANADA

NH

RAINBOW LAKE

This hike is somewhat ambitious for an overnight hike, but will reward you richly for your effort. If you don't have time to fit in the entire round-trip, you could camp at Hurd Brook Lean-to and just go to Rainbow Ledges or even Rainbow Lake the next day. Along either outing, you'll find views of Katahdin and the surrounding lake country as you climb over Rainbow Ledges. The destination is a campsite above Rainbow Lake, where the wild, piercing cry of the loon can often be heard. Optional side trips produce additional awe-inspiring views of Katahdin. This hike is at the northern end of the One Hundred Mile Wilderness, which stretches from Abol Bridge to Monson.

THE HIKE

The hike begins at Abol (short for Aboljackamegassic, Abenaki for "bare of trees") Bridge on the West Branch of the Penobscot River. The views of Katahdin from the bridge are the first of many fine vistas along this hike. Hiking south along the A.T., work your way over bog bridges, through a swampy area, and at mile 3.5, arrive at Hurd Brook Lean-to, where water is available.

From Hurd Brook Lean-to, the Trail soon begins to climb Rainbow Ledges, gaining about 750 feet in elevation over the next 2 miles. About 2.5 miles from the lean-to, you will reach the high point of the Ledges-

enjoy more excellent views of Katahdin. Hike another 1.6 miles to Rainbow Lake.

The opportunity to take a side trip to another vista appears 1.7 miles after reaching the lake. The Rainbow Mountain Trail ascends to the left for 1.1 miles. A major forest fire in the early part of the twentieth century created large open areas on the summit, providing you with excellent views of the surrounding countryside.

Continuing on the A.T., your destination for the night, Rainbow Spring Campsite, is on a short side trail to the left 1.7 miles from the intersection with Rainbow Mountain Trail. The spring is just below the A.T.

If you are feeling energetic, you could walk another 1.8 miles to the west end of Rainbow Lake for an additional view of Katahdin from the dam located along a short side trail. Return to the campsite to spend the night.

Return north via the A.T. to Abol Bridge.

TRAILHEAD DIRECTIONS

From Millinocket, travel 16 miles on Baxter Park Road to the turn for Baxter State Park. Instead of turning to the right to go to the Park, follow the main road and drive 4 miles to Abol Bridge. You can arrange to park your car in the campground at the bridge by talking to the camp's owner.

NAHMAKANTA LAKE
TO ABOL BRIDGE

A short float-plane flight from Millinocket, brings you to the trailhead for this wilderness hike. The trip covers the top quarter of the One Hundred Mile Wilderness, which stretches from Abol Bridge south to Monson. Nahmakanta Lake offers good swimming at several points near the A.T. The lake's wild surroundings make the cold swim all the more enjoyable. The only two climbs along the route—Nesuntabunt Mountain and Rainbow Ledges—have some steep sections, but are relatively easy and reward you with good views of Katahdin and the surrounding lake country.

THE HIKE

This overnight trip begins with a plane ride from Millinocket Lake. The hike begins at the south end of Nahmakanta Lake. The A.T. stays near the shore of the lake for 2.1 miles. Cross Wadleigh Stream at mile 2.5, and reach Wadleigh Stream Lean-to in another 0.1 mile. Water for the lean-to is available from the stream.

From the lean-to, hike 1.9 miles to the summit of Nesuntabunt Mountain. There are no views from the summit, but a short side trail leads to a rock ledge with fine views of Nahmakanta Lake and Katahdin. Descend 1.1 miles to the base of the mountain and continue 0.75 mile to Crescent Pond, which the Trail skirts for 0.6 mile. After leaving Crescent Pond, you will reach a logging bridge over Pollywog Stream in 1.4 miles, and Rainbow Stream in another 0.4 mile.

For the next 2 miles, the Trail follows Rainbow Stream, which offers several swimming holes. Just before crossing the stream, you will reach Rainbow Stream Lean-to. Water for the lean-to is available from the stream. The lean-to, one of two suggested campsites for this hike, is at mile 10.7. Continue on the A.T. for another 2 miles to the west end of Rainbow Lake and an excellent view of Katahdin. From here, hike 1.8 miles to Rainbow Lake Spring, a ten-foot wide spring on a short side trail to the left.

The Rainbow Spring Campsite is located on a short side trail to the right. After passing the spring, the A.T. continues to follow the shore of Rainbow Lake for another 3.4 miles and then begins to climb Rainbow Ledges. The highest point of the Ledges is reached 1.6 miles after you leave the lake. Several points along Rainbow Ledges afford excellent views of Katahdin.

From the high point along the Ledges, hike 2.5 miles to Hurd Brook Lean-to. Water is available from the brook. From Hurd Brook, hike 3.5 miles of often boggy trail to Abol Bridge on the West Branch of the Penobscot River. Return transportation should be arranged with the Air Service when you set up your flight.

TRAILHEAD DIRECTIONS

To make arrangements for the flight, contact Katahdin Air Service in Millinocket Lake, at (207) 723-8378 or (888)-742-5527. They offer reasonably priced flights to a number of points along the Trail in Maine, including Nahmakanta Lake.

Where and how to meet up with your flight can be arranged when you call the Katahdin Air Service.

COOPER POND TO NAHMAKANTA STREAM

MODERATE

15.8 MILES TRAVERSE

The ponds, lakes, and streams of Maine are some of its most beautiful places, and the A.T. and several short side trails along this hike enable you to experience all three. This is some of the easiest walking in the entire One Hundred Mile Wilderness, with just minor ups and downs. The most extended climb is over Potaywadjo Ridge— and it is only a little more than 300 feet worth of elevation gain spread out over a mile.

Possible campsites abound, but two of the most beautiful also happen to be sites designated by the Maine Appalachian Trail Club. Amidst the shade of a red pine grove, Antlers Campsite is located upon a somewhat narrow strip of land jutting into Lower Jo-Mary Lake, providing a great place to sit and watch the golden glow of a sunrise or pink hue of a sunset spread across the lake surface. Nahmakanta Stream Campsite is situated close to the tumbling waters of its namesake.

One of the most thrilling things that may happen on this journey is to turn a corner of the Trail just in time to catch a bull moose raising its head out of a pond. You might even hear it before you actually see it, as gallons upon gallons of liquid roll off a massive set of antlers, drip down the muscular neck, and splash loudly back into the water. During the summer, a moose's

favorite food is aquatic vegetation, such as water lilies and pondweeds, so you might also see a long strand of foliage hanging from its mouth.

THE HIKE

Follow the A.T. north. To enjoy the first of the ponds, take the side trail to the right at 1.3 miles and go another 0.2 mile to the north shore of Cooper Pond. Return to the A.T., continue north, and cross a gravel road over Cooper Brook at 3 miles. You may see signs of beaver near where you cross a number of outlet streams for Mud Pond at 3.3 miles.

So that you may appreciate the scenery around Antlers Campsite, take the side trail to the right at 4.6 miles for 300 feet to the campsite and point of land overlooking Lower Jo-Mary Lake. Return to the A.T and continue north, passing by the Potaywadjo Ridge Trail to the left at 6.2 miles. (This optional side trail rises for 1 mile to open ledges for views of Jo-Mary Mountain and several nearby lakes.) Take the side trail to the right at 6.4 miles and go 100 feet to a good swimming spot along a beach of Lower Jo-Mary Lake.

Back on the A.T., gradually rise and then descend to Potaywadjo Spring Lean-to at 8.2 miles. As someone once wrote in the shelter's register, the spring "is a true joy to all hikers." Gallons of water bubble out of the ground and into the 15-foot spring pool.

Cross Twitchell Brook at 8.7 miles and do not miss taking the short side trail (less than 100 feet) at 8.8 miles to the shore of Pemanumcook Lake and one of the most inspiring views of Katahdin in all of Maine. This is the first good look many northbound thru-hikers get of their final destination as the mountain rises dramatically in the distance, with the blue lake water in the foreground.

Return to the A.T., continue north, and ford a tributary of Nahmakanta Stream at 10.9 miles and Tumbledown Dick Stream at 12 miles. Pass Nahmakanta Stream Campsite at 12.5 miles and Wood Rat's Spring at 15.1 miles. Your shuttled car waits alongside the gravel road at 15.8 miles. Nah-makanta Lake is just another 0.3 mile north along the Trail if you wish to take in one more body of water before heading home.

TRAILHEAD DIRECTIONS

Drive south from Millinocket on Maine 11 for approximately 13 miles (or 18 miles north from Brownville Junction) and turn onto gravel Jo-Mary Road. This is a private logging road, but you will be permitted access after you pay a fee at the tollgate. Drive for 24 miles to leave one car next to the A.T. crossing just south of Nahmakanta Lake. Drive back toward the gate for 12 miles and leave the other car at the Trail crossing close to the bridge over Cooper Brook. Expect to spend quite a bit of time accomplishing this car shuttle.

BARREN—
CHAIRBACK RANGE

STRENUOUS

16.5 MILES
TRAVERSE

This rough and rocky mountain range has a lot to offer. You'll be traversing the five peaks of the Barren-Chairback Range in the One Hundred Mile Wilderness, which stretches from Abol Bridge near Baxter State Park south to Monson. In this section, the A.T. is crossed only by logging roads. Short side trails lead to three mountaintop ponds: Cloud, West Chairback, and East Chairback.

The elevation changes considerably between peaks and gaps along the range, a net gain in elevation of nearly 4,000 feet no matter which direction you hike. The Barren-Chairback Range is for experienced hikers looking for a wilderness trek.

Because this hike is a traverse, it will require either a drop-off/pick-up, shuttle, or two vehicles.

The Hike

From the parking lot on the St. Regis Logging Road, take the side trail 0.2 mile north to the A.T., turn left to follow it south, and cross the logging road at 0.7 mile. Immediately begin climbing Chairback Mountain. The trail ascends steadily for 1.2 miles before you reach a 0.25-mile side trail that leads to East Chairback Pond. From the junction with the pond side trail, hike 2.2 miles, crossing several ridges and then ascending sharply to the summit of Chairback Mountain (elevation 2,219 feet).

From the rocky, open summit of Chairback Mountain, enjoy noteworthy views of White Cap and the surrounding lakes and ponds. Hike 0.5 mile down Chairback Mountain to Chairback Gap Lean-to located in the gap between Chairback and Columbus Mountains. Water is available from a spring. From the lean-to, climb 0.5 mile to the top of Columbus Mountain (elevation 2,326 feet). The trail crosses a rocky viewpoint near the summit and then descends for 1.3 miles to a gap where an old tote road leads 0.25 mile to West Chairback Pond.

From the gap, a 0.6-mile climb brings you to Monument Cliff at the top of Third Mountain (elevation 2,061 feet), and another 2.5 miles will bring you over the top of Fourth Mountain (elevation 2,383 feet). After leaving this tree-covered peak, hike 2.1 miles to the side trail for Cloud Pond Lean-to. The 0.25-mile side trail leads to where the shelter sits on a small rise overlooking the lovely wilderness pond for which it is named. This is our favorite of the three shelters in the range. There is a spring along the side trail on the way to the shelter.

Continuing on the A.T. from the shelter side trail, hike 0.9 mile to the summit of Barren Mountain (elevation 2,670 feet), the fifth, and last, peak you'll encounter on the Barren-Chairback Range. Enjoy the fine 360-degree view of the surrounding area. From Barren Mountain, descend 1.8 miles to Barren Ledges where you'll find fine views of Lake Onawa and Boarstone Mountain. In another 1.3 miles, you will reach the 0.1-mile side trail that leads to Long Pond Stream Lean-to. Water is available from the stream.

From the lean-to side trail, hike for 0.1 mile to the short side trail to Slugundy Gorge and Falls. On the A.T., continue another 0.7 mile to ford Long Pond Stream (about knee deep). Take care, because the rocks can be quite slick and the streambed is uneven in places. After crossing the stream, you will reach the end of the hike, and your shuttled car, on the Long Pond Stream Tote Road.

Trailhead Directions

Access to the northern end of the hike is through the Katahdin Iron Works Gate. From Brownville Junction, take Maine 11 for 5.5 miles to Katahdin Iron Works Road. From here, it is 7 miles to the Katahdin Iron Works Gate. (There might be a fee.) After passing through the gate, take your first right and your next left onto the St. Regis Logging Road. Leave your car in the parking area 6.7 miles from the Katahdin Iron Works Gate.

To reach the southern end of the hike, turn right onto Elliotsville Road about a half mile northwest of Monson and make sure to stay to the left about 8 to 9 miles later after the Elliotsville Road crosses Big Wilson Stream. Almost 3 miles later, turn left onto Long Pond Stream Tote Road and follow it 1.5 miles to the A.T.

LITTLE WILSON FALLS

MODERATE

15.8 MILES
TRAVERSE

L ike the Cooper Pond to Nahmakanta Lake hike, this outing takes you across some of the lower elevations of the A.T.'s traverse through Maine, passing by several ponds and streams. A number of slate ridges and corresponding valleys cause you to negotiate quite a few ups and downs along the way, with some of them being quite steep. However, none of the elevation changes last for any great length.

With a 60-foot drop, Little Wilson Falls is considered by many to be the highest falls on the A.T. It is certainly one of the highest in Maine. Deep pools at its base are inviting swimming holes, but be careful if you decide to take a dip as you will need to drop almost 100 feet into the deep slate canyon to reach the water.

The Hike

Follow the A.T. north, ford Goodell Brook in 0.1 mile and cross the Old Stage Road in another 0.8 mile. At one time, a portion of the A.T. followed this roadway, which was the stagecoach route to Greenville, during the 1800s. During wet weather (which can be often in Maine), the road can become a sloppy, boggy, mucky mess to walk upon. Pass by Bell Pond at 1.2 miles, and a nice vista from the open ridgeline at 1.6 miles.

A short side trail at 1.9 miles leads right to Lily Pond, while Leeman Brook Lean-to is situated above the ravine at 3 miles, where the A.T. crosses the brook. Cross the outlet stream of North Pond at 3.8 miles and walk close to Mud Pond at 5.2 miles. Rise over Bear Pond Ledge and descend to Little Wilson Falls at 6.6 miles.

Ford Little Wilson Stream at 6.8 miles and make use of a long beaver dam to continue on your way at 7.1 miles. Cross over another slate ridge at 7.7 miles. The memorial marker for John F. Kennedy's gravesite in Arlington National Cemetery is made of this same type of slate and was quarried not too far from here.

Ford Big Wilson Stream at 9.7 miles. If the water is too high, you will either have to make this the turn-around point of your hike or walk 1.5 miles downstream to a roadway bridge and return upstream on the opposite bank.

Continue on the A.T. past Big Wilson Stream, and hike 0.3 mile to cross the railroad tracks of the Canadian Pacific Railway. This is the only active rail line the A.T. crosses in Maine, so as the Appalachian Trail Guide to Maine says, "Stop, look, and listen!" The short side trail to the Wilson Valley Lean-to is a short 0.4-mile walk north of the railroad tracks.

Return via the A.T. to the south.

Trailhead Directions

A parking area for the A.T. is located on Maine 15, 3.5 miles north of Monson.

MOXIE BALD MOUNTAIN, BALD MOUNTAIN, AND HORSESHOE CANYON

MODERATE

18.6 MILES
TRAVERSE

This picturesque hike gets a moderate rating because of the more than 1,500-foot climb of Moxie Bald Mountain (elevation 2,629 feet). Most of the elevation is gained in 2 miles, but the 360-degree view makes the ascent worthwhile. There are also two large ponds on the hike—at the onset of the hike and at the recommended campsite. Moxie (Indian for "dark water") Pond and Bald Mountain Pond offer great opportunities for swimming.

Good swimming is also available during the 5-mile walk along the West Branch of the Piscataquis River, which flows by the slate walls of Horseshoe Canyon. Numerous waterfalls and a grove of large white pine trees add to the beauty of the outing.

There are several stream fordings on this hike, including a crossing of Baker Stream, the confluence of West Branch of Piscataquis River and Bald Mountain Stream, and East Branch of Piscataquis River. Be careful crossing these wide waterways. If the water is too high to ford Baker Stream, there is a double-cable crossing available 0.1 mile downstream. For some people, the cable crossing is trickier than the ford, so use it only in extreme weather conditions.

An option: if you do not have two cars to do a shuttle or are short on time, you could hike out just to Moxie Bald Lean-To, enjoy the night, and return the way you came. This route is a round-trip journey of 13.8 miles.

THE HIKE

To begin this hike, walk a few feet down the road and follow the A.T. north as it fords Baker Stream at 0.1 mile. The pathway begins a slow and gradual ascent of Moxie Bald Mountain. In the next mile, you will pass beneath a power transmission right-of-way before crossing Joe's Hole Brook at 1.2 miles. The Bald Mountain Brook Campsite is near the Bald Mountain Brook crossing at 2.6 miles, while a side trail at 2.8 miles leads right for 0.1 mile to the Bald Mountain Brook Lean-to.

The A.T. begins to ascend steeply up the face of Moxie Bald Mountain. At 4.2 miles, you will reach the junction with the blue-blazed trail that bypasses the summit. This 0.5-mile trail can be used to avoid the summit in foul weather. Take the A.T. for another 0.4 mile to the summit of Moxie Bald Mountain, and enjoy the 360-degree view. Look west to the Bigelow Mountain Range and northeast to the Barren-Chairback Range. On especially clear days, you can see Katahdin.

Descend north from the summit toward the sag in the ridge, and follow the ridge toward the north peak of Moxie Bald. At 5.1 miles, you will reach the junction with the northern end of the Trail that bypasses the summit. Water is available from a spring 0.1 mile down this blue-blazed trail. Before descending steeply toward Bald Mountain Pond, you will reach the junction of the side trail that leads 0.75 mile to the north peak of Moxie Bald. This trail crosses many open ledges with great views, and it is strongly recommended that you take this optional side trip. The north peak also features outstanding blueberry picking in season.

Continuing on the A.T, you will cross a small brook and reach the short side trail at 6.9 miles to Moxie Bald Lean-to, which sits on the shore of Bald Mountain Pond. Along the A.T., you will ford Bald Mountain Stream at 9 miles, and cross Marble Brook at 12.4. Ford the confluence of West Branch of Piscataquis River and Bald Mountain Stream at 12.7 miles as you enter the confines of Horseshoe Canyon. Picataquis is Abenaki for "at the river branch."

Side trails of 0.1 mile in length to the Horseshoe Canyon Lean-to are passed at 15.7 miles and 15.9 miles. Ford the East Branch of the Piscataquis River at 18.1

miles, and walk along the bed of the former Bangor and Aroostock Railroad for a short distance around 18.4 miles. Make a quick ascent and turn right onto the Shirley-Blanchard Road to come to your shuttled car at 18.6 miles.

TRAILHEAD DIRECTIONS

The Shirley-Blanchard Road comes in contact with the A.T. 1.3 miles north of the main crossroads in Blanchard. A parking area is 0.1 mile south of the trail crossing.

To reach the southern trailhead of this hike, drive Maine 16 northeast for 0.8 mile from US 201 in Bingham, turn left onto the Scott Paper Company gravel road, and follow it about to 15 miles to the A.T. crossing. Parking is in a small area just to the south of the A.T.

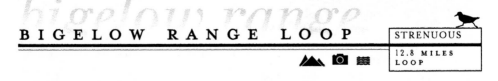

BIGELOW RANGE LOOP

STRENUOUS

12.8 MILES
LOOP

This short, but challenging, overnight hike traverses a section of the Bigelow Range and is one of the best wilderness hikes in a state known for its wilderness trails. The A.T. ascends Bigelow Mountain to a wonderful mountain tarn—Horns Pond—at more than 3,000 feet in elevation. From Horns Pond, the A.T. ascends South

Horn and the West Peak of Bigelow, where there is an awe-inspiring view of Flagstaff Lake and numerous surrounding mountains, including Sugarloaf and the Crocker Mountains to the southwest.

The return trip on the Firewarden's Trail and along Stratton Brook Pond Road makes this entire outing a nice two-day trip.

A side trip to the summit of Avery Peak is an optional 0.75-mile hike that will richly reward you for your efforts. Like the West Peak, Avery Peak boasts a commanding 360-degree view of the surrounding mountains and lakes.

The hike is located almost entirely in the Bigelow State Preserve. The Preserve is a 33,000-acre wilderness area the people of Maine set aside by a 3,000-vote margin in a general election in the 1970s. Prior to the legislation, commercial interests had hoped to develop the Bigelow Range as a ski area. Led by the Friends of Bigelow, the Maine Appalachian Trail Club and numerous other conservation groups helped force the referendum that saved the range from future development.

The Hike

From the trailhead on Stratton Brook Pond Road, hike north on the A.T. In 0.2 mile, cross Stratton Brook and begin the climb of Bigelow, which starts gradually, but gets steeper. Pass by Cranberry Stream Campsite at 1.1 miles and, at 2.4 miles, the Bigelow Range Trail, which leads left 4.6 miles to Stratton Village. Continue on the A.T., where a short side trail at 3.3 miles goes to an overlook of the Crocker and Sugarloaf Mountains to the south. Another viewpoint, right on the A.T. at 3.5 miles, looks onto Little Bigelow, the Horns, Sugarloaf, and the Crockers. An additional view of Horns Pond is available from one more side trail at 4 miles. Descend on the A.T., pass by the junction with the Horns Pond Trail at 4.1 miles, and in another 0.2 mile, arrive at the twin Horns Pond Shelters. There are several tent sites nearby, and water is available from a spring in the camping area. The solar privy was built to minimize hikers' impact on the pond's ecosystem.

From the lean-tos at Horns Pond, climb 0.4 mile to a side trail to North Horn and another 0.2 mile along the A.T. to the open summit of South Horn (elevation 3,805 feet). Descend to follow the main crest of the mountain before rising once again, this time to the top of the West Peak of Bigelow (elevation 4,145) at 6.9 miles. The 360-degree view from the rocky summit is tremendous. Ridgeline after ridgeline march off to the southwest. Close by, view Crocker and Sugarloaf; on a clear day, Mount Washington in New Hampshire. Down below, view Flagstaff Lake, which was formed in the 1940s. Remember, the plants on the summit are fragile; stick to the Trail.

Descend steeply for 0.3 mile to Bigelow Col (where designated campsites are available) and the junction with the Firewarden's Trail. (From the Col, there is an optional 0.75-mile hike to Avery Peak, a rewarding side trip.) For the return portion of this loop, hike down the Firewarden's Trail from the Col. The first 0.75 mile is very steep; afterwards the Trail descends more moderately. Pass by the junction with the Horns Pond Trail 2.3 miles after leaving the Col. Hike another 2.3 miles to Stratton Brook Pond Road. Follow the road for about a mile back to the trailhead.

Trailhead Directions

Stratton Brook Pond Road is about 4 miles south of Stratton, on Maine 27. Turn left on Stratton Brook Pond Road and drive 1 mile to the trailhead.

SADDLEBACK RANGE

STRENUOUS

23.9 MILES
TRAVERSE

▲▲ 📷 ≈

Western Maine offers some excellent hiking opportunities, but the Saddleback Mountain Range heads the list, boasting a 3-mile above–tree line section with outstanding views. Before you climb Saddleback Mountain, The Horn, and Saddleback Junior, you will pass Piazza Rock, an overhanging rock that juts out from a cliff. You will also walk near the shores of Ethel and Eddy Ponds. From Saddleback Junior's treeless peak, there are views in all directions of the surrounding western Maine wilderness. You will ford the cold, clear waters of Orbeton Stream before you climb Lone and Spaulding Mountains. Maine's second highest peak—Sugarloaf Mountain—is located on a 0.6-mile optional side trail. The trail then descends sharply to the sometimes tricky ford of the South Branch of the Carrabassett River.

The ridge between Spaulding and Sugarloaf Mountains was the last section of the Appalachian Trail to be built. When a Civilian Conservation Corps crew blazed this section of trail in 1937, it completed the more than 2,000-mile Appalachian Trail from Maine to Georgia.

This is a strenuous hike and should not be taken lightly. The above–tree line sections leave the unprepared hiker exposed to the elements; weather changes quickly often in these mountains. The Saddleback Range offers no protection from lightning or severe rain or snow. Follow the Boy Scout motto and "be prepared." Avoid this hike in inclement weather.

Though this can be done as an overnight hike, it is easier if done in three days. By setting up cars at both ends, you can hike the 1.4 miles to Piazza Rock Lean-to and*f* then continue to walk the remainder of this hike the following two days.

THE HIKE

From the trailhead on Maine 4, follow the A.T. north and cross Sandy River on a footbridge in 0.1 mile. From Sandy River, hike 1.7 miles to Piazza Rock Lean-to. Water is available from the nearby stream. A short side trail leads to Piazza Rock.

After leaving the lean-to, the A.T. leads 0.9 mile to Ethel Pond and another 1 mile to the outlet of Moose and Deer Pond near Eddy Pond, which sits at the base of the climb up Saddleback. (Note that this is the last sure water source for 5.9 miles.) The trail ascends steeply up the west side of the mountain, gaining well over 1,000 feet in elevation during the first mile. Rise above–tree line at 4.7 miles and reach the open summit of Saddleback (elevation 4,120 feet) at 5.7 miles, with outstanding views of the western Maine mountains. Descend to the gap between Saddleback and the Horn, and then ascend the Horn steeply, reaching the summit (elevation 4,041 feet) at 7.3 miles. Just 0.4 mile from the summit of the Horn, the Trail drops below tree line again, continuing to descend sharply off the Horn and reaching the short, steep climb up Saddleback Junior. The distance between the Horn and the treeless summit of Saddleback Junior (elevation 3,655 feet) is 2 miles. After enjoying Saddleback Junior's fine 360-degree vista, descend, and reach Poplar Ridge Lean-to in 1.4 miles. Water is available from the nearby stream.

From the lean-to, hike 0.5 mile to the high point on Poplar Ridge, and descend steeply for 0.5 mile, losing 1,000 feet in elevation. Reach the ford of Orbeton Stream, 2.7 miles from Poplar Ridge Lean-to. The trail climbs steeply and then moderately out of Orbeton Stream Valley and reaches the summit of Lone Mountain (elevation 3,280 feet) at 16.5 miles. Arrive at the junction with the side trail to Mount Abraham (elevation 4,043 feet) in 1.1 miles. If you allow three days for this hike, you may want to add a trip to Abraham, 3.4 miles round-trip. There are outstanding views from both the mountain and the ridge.

Continue following the A.T. and reach the short side trail to Spaulding Mountain Lean-to in 1.1 miles. Water is available from a spring near the shelter. From the lean-to, hike 0.8 mile to the side trail that leads to Spaulding Mountain. It is just 0.1 mile along the side trail to Spaulding's tree-covered summit (elevation 3,988 feet). Continue following the A.T. and reach the side trail to Sugarloaf Mountain (elevation 4,237 feet) in 2.1 miles. It is 0.6 mile along that route to the top of Sugarloaf.

Continue following the A.T. for 1.4 miles to the top of an open ravine. It is more than 500 feet to the forest below. Descend, sometimes steeply, for 0.8 mile to the South Branch of the Carrabassett River. This ford can be difficult, particularly after heavy rain. The hike ends, after another 0.1 mile, at Caribou Valley Road.

TRAILHEAD DIRECTIONS

The trailhead on ME 4 is 9 miles south of Rangeley. To reach the northern trailhead, drive eastward from Stratton, on Maine 27 for about 8 miles to turn right onto (possibly) unsigned gravel Caribou Valley Road (this is also 1 mile west of the Sugarloaf USA access road). The conditions of Caribou Valley Road vary greatly from time to time and it may not always be possible to drive the 4.2 miles to the A.T. crossing.

HIKE OF THE
FIVE PONDS

MODERATE

13.6 MILES
TRAVERSE
INCLUDES THE
ROADWALK ON
MAINE 17

The ponds of Maine are beautiful, and on this hike you experience not just one, but five. The flora and fauna are also representative of the state. The journey begins in a hardwood forest with a floor that is dotted with trout lily and spring beauty just as the weather begins to warm after winter. At a bit higher elevation, in the spruce and fir forest, be on the lookout for a spruce grouse or Canada jay. In New England, the spruce grouse is often called a partridge. The Canada jay has earned the nickname "camp robber" because it has been known to be brave enough to boldly hop into camp and make off with bits of food from a hungry hiker's plate. Moose and loons are often seen in or around all five ponds.

The great scenery and gentle terrain—only a couple of short uphills—make this the perfect place to break friends into the pleasures of hiking without introducing them to the rigors of a more rugged topography. Swimming opportunities abound, as do possible campsites in exceptionally beautiful locations.

THE HIKE

Walk northward along Maine 17 for 0.5 mile to a highway turnout overlooking the Bemis Range and Mooselookmeguntic Lake. Turn right and follow the A.T. to the north, reaching the forested summit of Spruce Mountain at 1.3 miles, and walking near the north shore of Moxie Pond at 2.1 miles.

Rise to an overlook of Long Pond on Bates Ledge at 3 miles and come to a sandy beach along the pond's edge at 3.9 miles. Sabbath Day Pond with its waterside lean-to

is passed at 4.2 miles. Cross an old fire road at 4.7 miles, and climb to the high point on the landscape at 6.4 miles. Little Swift River Pond Campsite is located close to its namesake at 8.8 miles. A spring situated near the pond can be found about 30 yards from the Trail.

Cross Chandler Mill Stream, the outlet of a boreal bog, at 10 miles. Most of the bogs in Maine are the result of glaciers. Some bogs began as embedded ice that melted to leave a lake, some were basins gouged out by moving glaciers, and still others were produced as the glaciers receded and deposited tons of rock and mud that impeded the flow of water.

Walk close to South Pond at 11.5 miles, the Trail will soon rise somewhat steeply for a short distance to a view from the high point at 12.5 miles. Descend and reach Maine 4 at 13.6 miles.

TRAILHEAD DIRECTIONS

For the southern trailhead, there is a parking area for hikers on ME 17 about 0.5 mile south of the A.T. and about 25.5 miles north of Rumford (and just past the Bemis Stream Trailhead).

The northern trailhead on ME 4 is 9 miles south of Rangeley.

BEMIS RANGE LOOP

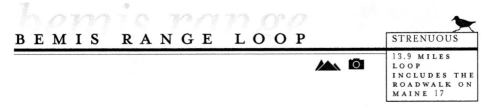

STRENUOUS

13.9 MILES
LOOP
INCLUDES THE
ROADWALK ON
MAINE 17

This relatively difficult hike features the four open peaks of the Bemis Range and the ledges that connect them. You hike the A.T. for 7.3 miles and connect with the Bemis Stream Trail for the last 5.6 miles. At the beginning of the hike, there is a 0.5-mile roadwalk from the parking area at the trailhead of the Bemis Valley Trail to the Appalachian Trail. In season, blueberries are abundant along the ledges; on clear days, there are excellent views of the Rangeley lakes to the north as well as most of the major peaks of Northwest Maine.

THE HIKE

After parking close to the Bemis Stream Trailhead on Maine 17, hike 0.5 mile up the road to its junction with the A.T. The A.T. crosses ME 17 at a turnout, which offers views of Mooselookmeguntic Lake, and the Bemis Range. Follow the A.T. south to descend immediately into the Bemis Valley.

At 1.3 miles, Bemis Stream runs along the valley's floor and can be difficult to ford when the water is high. Only 0.2 mile after fording the stream, you will cross a gravel road built over a former line of the Rumford and Rangeley Lakes Railroad, abandoned in the 1930s. Begin to ascend the Bemis Range.

In about 0.1 mile, pass a small spring and continue the ascent to the first of many open ledges and knobs. A large cairn marks the First Peak of the Bemis Range (elevation

2,604 feet) at 2.7 miles. Just under a mile later, the Second Peak is reached (elevation 2,915 feet).

Continue along the A.T. and you will reach the Bemis Mountain Lean-to in another 1.5 miles. The lean-to is located in a sag, and water is available from a nearby spring. Consider spending the night here, leaving yourself an 8.3-mile hike for the following day. If you go on, stock up on water because this spring is the only sure water source in the Bemis Range.

From the shelter, hike less than 0.5 mile to the summit of Third Peak of Bemis Range (elevation 3,115 feet). The main summit of Bemis is made up of two peaks-the East and the West. In 1.2 miles, you will top East Peak (elevation 3,532 feet) and 0.1 mile later, West Peak (elevation 3,592 feet). The A.T. then descends from the west peak into the saddle between Bemis and Elephant Mountain.

In 1 mile, you will reach the junction of the A.T. with the Bemis Steam Trail. Take the Bemis Stream Trail and descend, crossing the waterway twice before returning to ME 17 at 13.9 miles.

TRAILHEAD DIRECTIONS

There is a parking area for hikers on ME 17, about 0.5 mile south of the A.T. and about 25.5 miles north of Rumford (and just past the Bemis Stream Trailhead).

THE BALDPATES

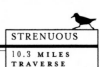

The Baldpates and the spectacular water-falls of Dunn Notch are the outstanding features of this trip. The net elevation gain of 3,300 feet over rough terrain creates a tough but short hike for experienced back-packers. Like many peaks in this wilderness state, the Baldpates offer incredible views of the mountains and lakes of western Maine. The 1,000-foot cliffs at Grafton Notch on Maine 26 are outstanding.

THE HIKE

This hike begins at East B Hill Road, which also connects to the northwest with ME 26 near Upton Village. From East B Hill Road, the A.T. crosses a brook and heads south and west toward Dunn Notch.

Reach Dunn Notch in less than a mile and cross the West Branch of the Ellis River. A side trail of 0.2 mile leads to the falls. Downstream from the Trail crossing is a 60-foot double waterfall that spills into a deep gorge. A road on the south bank of the river provides access to the bottom of the falls. You can also follow the river upstream to the upper falls, which spill into a small gorge.

From the falls, the A.T. ascends steeply out of the notch's south rim, and reaches the top of the rim in 0.2 mile. The trail ascends gradually for the next 3 miles before swinging onto the northeast ridge of Surplus Mountain.

At mile 4.5, reach your destination for the day—Frye Notch Lean-to and the adjacent Frye Brook.

Only 1.2 miles beyond the lean-to, rise above–tree line on the shoulder of Little Bald-pate Mountain. It is another 0.1 mile to the peak of Little Baldpate. Continue your ascent up the Baldpates and at mile 6.3 arrive on the open summit of East Baldpate (elevation 3,812 feet), with a grand 360-degree vista.

The trail heads into the sag between the East and West Peaks of Baldpate (there is a small canyon at the bottom of the sag) and arrives on the partially open summit of West Baldpate (elevation 3,680 feet) after nearly a mile.

Descending from the West Peak toward Grafton Notch, you will pass by the Bald-pate Lean-to next to a small stream at mile 8. In another 1.5 miles, you will reach the junction with the Table Rock Trail, which leads just over 0.5 mile to Table Rock that overlooks the sheer cliffs that fall away into Grafton Notch. The Table Rock Trail meets up with the A.T. at the bottom of the notch near ME 26 in another 0.7 mile.

Reach ME 26 at mile 10.3.

TRAILHEAD DIRECTIONS

For the northern trailhead, the A.T. crossing is on East B Hill Road, 8 miles northwest of Andover. East B Hill Road also connects to the northwest with ME 26 near Upton Village. The southern trailhead is in Grafton Notch, 12 miles north of US 2 on ME 26 (18 miles from Bethel).

MAHOOSUC RANGE

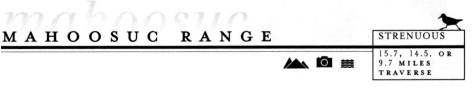

The Mahoosuc Range is the most rugged section of A.T. in the state of Maine. A lot of elevation is gained and lost. The mountains in this chain are all more than 3,500 feet in elevation. Because you will be hiking along the crest of the ridge, water will be scarce. Be sure to carry plenty.

The treadway is often wet and rough, and the trails cross many boggy areas, high on the ridge and in the sags. Because these areas can get so muddy, many bog bridges have been installed to protect the delicate ecosystem. Please remain on these bridges.

The most outstanding feature of the Mahoosuc Range is Mahoosuc Notch. This deep cleft between Mahoosuc Arm and Fulling Mill Mountain is filled with enormous boulders that have fallen from the sheer cliffs on either side of the notch. Even in July, you can find ice in some of the caves formed by the boulders. The moss and boulders are slick and wet. Be careful. This is not the place to have an accident! Once you're down among the boulders, there is no way around them except over, under, and to either side. Although less than 1 mile in length, Mahoosuc Notch can take several hours to maneuver through. Be sure to allow for the extra time.

All three of these hikes begin and end on Success Pond Road and use side trails to get to and from the A.T. However, there are several miles between Speck Pond Trail and where it ends at Carlo Col, Goose Eye, and Mahoosuc Notch Trails, so it will be necessary to arrange a shuttle, drop-off/pick-up, or park two vehicles at the Trail's ends.

THE HIKES

To reach Carlo Col Trail (15.7 miles), hike 3.6 miles up the Speck Pond Trail to reach the campsite at Speck Pond, a mountain tarn between Old Speck and Mahoosuc Arm. A tarn is defined as a small mountain lake or pond, especially one found in a cirque, a rounded bowl carved out by glacial action. The Speck Pond Trail and A.T. join at the Speck Pond Campsite. From here, follow the A.T. sharply left and skirt the eastern side of Speck Pond. The A.T. follows the Appalachian Mountain Club's (AMC) Mahoosuc Trail along the crest of the ridge.

After crossing the outlet of Speck Pond, you will begin your ascent up Mahoosuc Arm (elevation 3,777 feet). Less than 1 mile after the junction with the Speck Pond Trail, the A.T. tops the open summit of Mahoosuc Arm. From here, descend gradually, then more steeply, over ledges into Mahoosuc Notch.

Before entering the notch, you will cross a brook, turn right, and head upstream along the Bull Branch of the Sunday River. The route through the notch is both difficult and dangerous: take care. Follow the white blazes through the notch for 1.1 miles, and at its western end, reach the junction of the Mahoosuc Notch Trail. The A.T. turns sharply left and begins its ascent of Fulling

Mill Mountain. The Mahoosuc Notch Trail descends out of the range to Success Pond Road 2.5 miles away. (This is where the Speck Pond Trail to Mahoosuc Notch Trail hike ends; a total of 9.7 miles.)

Continue on the A.T. and reach the crest of the South Peak of Fulling Mill Mountain (elevation 3,420 feet) in 1 mile. From here, turn right and descend, passing the side trail to Full Goose Shelter just past the bottom of the sag. There is a short side trail at the shelter that leads to water, a scarce commodity along this hike. Beyond the shelter side trail, the A.T. ascends steeply and then levels off a bit. One mile past the shelter, you will reach the summit of the North Peak of Goose Eye Mountain (elevation 3,6750 feet).

Turn left toward a long line of cairns, walk past the north fork of the Wright Trail in 1.1 miles and reach the summit of the East Peak of Goose Eye Mountain (elevation 3,794 feet) just 0.1 mile later. The south fork of the Wright Trail is 0.1 mile beyond the summit. Reach the junction with the Goose Eye Trail in another 0.3 mile. The Goose Eye Trail tops the summit of the West Peak of Goose Eye (elevation 3,854 feet) in 0.1 mile. Descend west off the range for 3.1 miles to Success Pond Road. (This is where the Speck Pond Trail to Goose Eye Trail hike ends; a total of 14.5 miles.)

The A.T. turns left, bypassing the west peak, and descending steeply into a sag. From the bottom of the sag, the A.T. ascends for 0.6 mile to the summit of Mount Carlo (elevation 3,565 feet). Then, the A.T. bears right, descends toward the Col ahead, and meets the junction with the Carlo Col Trail 0.4 mile later. Follow this trail for 0.3 mile to the Carlo Col Shelter. Hike another 2.3 miles on the Carlo Col Trail, descending off the range to the northwest, to Success Pond Road. (This is where the Success Pond Trail to Carlo Col Trail hike ends; a total of 15.7 miles.)

TRAILHEAD DIRECTIONS

Success Pond Road, which provides access to the trails used for all three hikes—Speck Pond, Mahoosuc Notch, Goose Eye and Carlo Col—can be reached from Berlin. From New Hampshire 16 in Berlin, cross the Androscoggin River on Cleveland Bridge (Unity Street), keep left, and pass traffic signals at 0.7 mile. The roadway swings right at 0.8 mile, crosses railroad tracks, and becomes Hutchins Street. The road turns sharp[y left at 1.6 miles and passes the James River mill yard.

Success Pond Road is the wide gravel road on the right (this will be 1.9 miles from NE 16). It is about 8 miles down Success Pond Road to the trailhead (on right) for both the Carlo Col and Goose Eye Trails; 11 miles to the trailhead (on right) for the Mahoosuc Notch Trail; and 12.5 miles to the trailhead (on right) for the Speck Pond Trail. If you pass Success Pond on the left, you have gone too far.

FROM THE MAHOOSUC RANGE ON THE MAINE BORDER, THE A.T. IN NEW HAMPSHIRE HEADS WEST OVER THE RUGGED CARTER-MORIAH/WILDCAT RANGE TO PINKHAM NOTCH. FROM PINKHAM NOTCH, THE TRAIL TRAVERSES THE NORTHERN PRESIDENTIAL RANGE WITH MILES OF ABOVE–TREE LINE TRAIL. THIS IS A VERY ROUGH AND REMOTE SECTION OF TRAIL. IN THE WHITE MOUNTAIN NATIONAL FOREST, WHICH ATTRACTS THOUSANDS OF VISITORS EACH YEAR, MANY HIKERS UNDERESTIMATE

New Hampshire

THE RUGGEDNESS OF THE TERRAIN. THE WEATHER CAN QUICKLY TURN SEVERE IN THESE HIGH ELEVATIONS; EVEN IF THE WEATHER IN THE VALLEYS IS EXPECTED TO BE NICE, BE PREPARED FOR THE WORST WHEN HIKING IN THE WHITES. MOUNT WASHINGTON AND OTHER PEAKS AND RIDGELINES CAN GET SNOW YEAR-ROUND.

AS THE A.T. CROSSES THE WHITE MOUNTAINS, IT GOES UP AND OVER SOME OF THE AREA'S BEST-KNOWN PEAKS, INCLUDING MOUNT MADISON, MOUNT WASHINGTON, MOUNT LAFAYETTE, FRANCONIA RIDGE, KINSMAN MOUNTAIN, AND MOUNT MOOSI-LAUKE. FROM THE WHITES, THE TRAIL CLIMBS MOUNT CUBE AND SMARTS MOUNTAIN ON THE WAY TO HANOVER. THE TRAIL GOES RIGHT THROUGH TOWN AND PASSES DARTMOUTH COLLEGE, HOME OF THE DARTMOUTH OUTING CLUB THAT MAINTAINS A PORTION OF THE TRAIL IN THIS AREA.

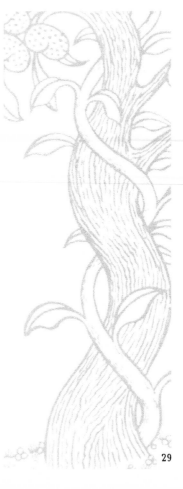

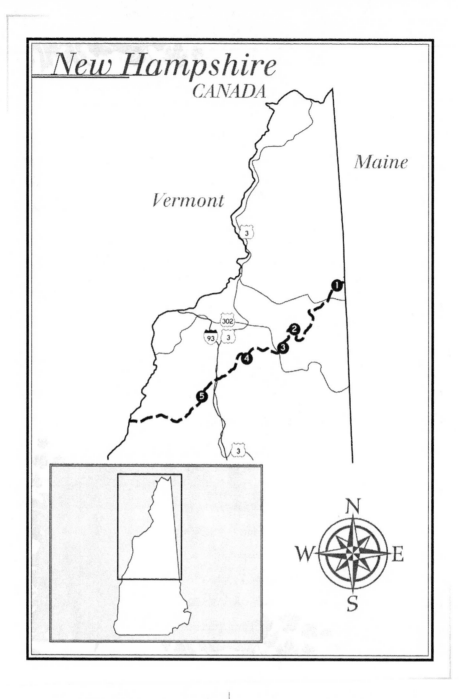

New Hampshire

CANADA

Maine

Vermont

GENTIAN POND

The highlights of this overnight hike are four mountain tarns. You will hike by Page Pond, Dream Lake, and Moss Pond before reaching Gentian Pond, where you can spend the night at the shelter or camp on the hill overlooking the pond.

This hike will also take you over the east summit of Mount Hayes (elevation 2,555 feet) where you'll find stunning views of the northern Presidentials and the Carter-Moriah Range. The peak is reached via a 0.2-mile side trail. This is a roller-coaster hike, but there are no major changes in elevation following the 3-mile climb to the east summit of Mount Hayes, during which you'll gain 1,500 feet.

THE HIKE

From the trailhead on Hogan Road, follow the A.T. (which runs along the Centennial Trail) north into the woods and begin ascending Mount Hayes. At mile 2.7, reach the east summit of Mount Hayes, and at mile 3.1, reach the Mahoosuc Trail (the Centennial Trail ends here). In order to obtain a vista, turn to the left and follow a section of the Mahoosuc Trail 0.2 mile to the peak of Mount Hayes (elevation 2,555 feet). Upon returning to the A.T., continue to follow it and the other portion of the Mahoosuc Trail as the route descends to the col between Mount Hayes and Cascade Mountain. Immediately begin a moderate ascent up Cascade Mountain.

At mile 5.4, reach the top of Cascade Mountain (elevation 2,631 feet). The Trail takes a hard left turn, continues along the top of the mountain, and begins the occasionally steep, 1.1 mile descent to Trident Col. The Trident Col Campsite is 0.1 mile via the side trail to the left.

Hike the A.T. 1 mile to Page Pond, climb to Wocket Ledge at mile 8.1, descend to walk beside Dream Lake, and continue to Moss Pond, the smallest of the four tarns along the hike, at mile 10.7. From Moss Pond, descend moderately to Gentian Pond. Water is available just upstream of the Trail where the A.T. crosses a creek on a footbridge prior to arriving at Gentian Pond. You will reach the Gentian Pond Shelter and Campsite at mile 11.4. A solar privy near the shelter is designed to lessen hikers' impact on the area. Return by way of the A.T. to the trailhead.

TRAILHEAD DIRECTIONS

From Gorham, drive 3.6 miles east on US 2, and turn left onto North Road. Note the white blazes along North Road as the A.T. follows the road on this section of trail. Turn left onto Hogan Road in 0.5 mile and travel another 0.25 mile down this gravel road. Parking is available where the Trail turns into the woods.

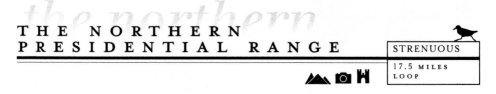

THE NORTHERN
PRESIDENTIAL RANGE

The A.T. is followed for all but 4.1 miles of this magnificent loop around the Northern Presidential Range of the White Mountains. The loop uses the Tuckerman Ravine Trail to descend from the summit of Mount Washington—the highlight of this hike—to Pinkham Notch. The Presidentials are the highest mountain group traversed by the A.T. north of Clingmans Dome (located in the Great Smoky Mountains National Park, North Carolina and Tennessee).

The Trail runs above–tree line for more than 8 miles of this outing. The tree line in the Presidential Range is at 4,200 feet, and above this elevation the only vegetation is krummholz (stunted spruce) and alpine plants, both extremely vulnerable to foot traffic. Please remain on the trails. Because of the potential for inclement weather in the Whites—rapidly arising storms with hurricane-force winds and freezing conditions—it is always a good idea to keep to the trails.

Mount Washington is said to have the worst weather in the world, producing record gusts of wind atop its 6,288-foot peak. In 1934, the weather observatory, established in 1870, recorded a wind velocity of 231 mph that has yet to be matched. Standing well above–tree line, Mount Washington, along with the rest of the Presidentials, forms an island of flora usually only found close to the arctic circle. Come prepared to throw on raingear and other layers of clothing at a moment's notice.

The first path to the summit was cut in 1819. The first summit house was built in 1852. The second summit house, the Tip Top, was built in 1853 and is still standing. It is open daily during season as a museum. The summit also features the Sherman Adams Building, which houses the weather observatory and its museum, as well as a snack bar, souvenir shop, post office, rest rooms, and telephones. The Mount Washington Auto Road (toll) climbs 8 miles from New Hampshire 16 to the summit. The world's first mountain-climbing railway, the Mount Washington Cog Railway, has been carrying tourists to the top of Washington since 1869. The 3.5-mile railroad climbs at a 37.4 percent grade, the steepest in the world.

If you intend to stay at one of the huts (as opposed to a tent site or shelter), you must make reservations through the Appalachian Mountain Club (AMC). Call (603) 466-2727 or write to Reservations, AMC, P. O. Box 298, Gorham, New Hampshire 03581. Fees are inexpensive for tent sites and shelters (close to $10 per person), but hut fees are around $90 per person, which includes lodging, breakfast, and dinner.

THE HIKE

You will start out on the A.T./Tuckerman Ravine Trail at Pinkham Notch, following this trail for a short distance before turning right onto the A.T./Old Jackson Road Trail. At mile 1.4, make a sharp left away from the old roadbed near a brook and begin to climb steeply.

You will soon pass the junction with Raymond Path (leading left across the mountain to Tuckerman Ravine Trail). Not long after the A.T. crosses a brook, you will pass the junction with the Nelson Crag Trail (leading left past Nelson Crag to the Mount Washington Auto Road).

At mile 1.7, you will cross the Mount Washington Auto Road at its two-mile post and take the A.T/Madison Gulf Trail into the Great Gulf Wilderness. In a few feet, a side trail leads right 0.1 mile to Lowe's Bald Spot and great views of the Northern Presidentials and the Carter-Moriah Range.

In another 0.5 mile, you will cross twin brooks and continue your ascent. At mile 4, the A.T./Madison Gulf Trail joins the Great Gulf Trail for a short distance. You will soon cross the West Branch of the Peabody River over a suspension bridge and ascend a ridge.

At mile 4.1, the Madison Gulf Trail turns left, while the A.T./Great Gulf Trail heads right to cross Parapet Brook. Shortly thereafter, come to the junction with the Osgood Cutoff Trail at mile 4.2. The A.T. now follows the Osgood Cutoff to the left, and comes to the intersection with the Osgood Trail at mile 4.8. The A.T. turns left onto the Osgood Trail (Osgood Campsite with the last sure water for 3 miles is to the right) and ascends steeply.

At mile 6.1, you will reach tree line on the crest of Osgood Ridge. For the next 8 miles or so, you will be above–tree line. Reach Osgood Junction at mile 6.8. The Daniel Webster Trail descends right, while Parapet Trail goes off to the left.

The A.T. continues up the ridge on the Osgood Trail, passing the intersection with the Howker Ridge Trail before reaching the summit of Mount Madison (elevation 5,363 feet) at mile 7.3. Watson Path descends right; the A.T. descends the southwest ridge of Mount Madison.

In another 0.5 mile, you will reach Madison Springs Hut. From the hut, the A.T. follows Gulfside Trail, soon crosses Snyder Brook, and ascends southwest. In 0.3 mile, you will reach the junction of the A.T. with the Air Line Trail to the right; a short distance further, the Air Line Trail leaves the A.T. to the left, climbing 0.8 mile to the summit of Mount Adams (elevation 5,798 feet). The A.T. continues to ascend gradually to the southwest.

At mile 8.7, reach Thunderstorm Junction. It is marked by a massive rock cairn more than ten feet high. Lowe's Path heads left 0.3 mile to the summit of Mount Adams. It also descends to the right to Gray Knob Cabin. Spur Trail descends north to Crag Camp Cabin; the Great Gully Trail descends into King Ravine. The A.T. continues along Gulfside Trail, passing a grassy area between Mount Adams and Mount Sam Adams.

In 0.3 mile, reach the northern intersection of the A.T. with Israel Ridge Path, which also leads to the summit of Mount Adams. At mile 9.3, reach the southern intersection where Israel Ridge Path descends 0.9 mile to The Perch Shelter. The A.T. continues ahead, following the narrow ridge between Castle Ravine on the right and Jefferson Ravine on the left.

In 0.7 mile, you will reach Edmands Col, where Randolph Path heads right 0.2 mile to Spaulding Spring, and Edmands Col Cutoff heads left, passing Gulfside Spring about 100 feet later. The A.T. continues along the eastern side of Mount Jefferson, passing the north end of the Jefferson Loop in 0.1 mile. The loop heads right for 0.3 mile to the summit of Mount Jefferson (elevation 5,715 feet).

Continuing along the eastern flank of the mountain, the A.T. soon reaches its intersection with Six Husbands Trail (left to Jefferson Ravine and Great Gulf Wilderness; right to the summit of Jefferson). In another

0.25 mile, the A.T. passes a smooth, grassy plateau known as Monticello Lawn. Jefferson Loop enters from the right.

The Cornice Trail descends to the right in another 0.25 mile, the Sphinx Trail to the left 0.5 mile later. Soon you will reach Clay-Jefferson Col, where the Mount Clay Loop heads left to the summit of Mount Clay (elevation 5,532 feet). Avoiding the summits, the graded A.T./Gulfside Trail continues along the western side of the ridge.

At mile 12.3, when you pass the junction of Jewell Trail, the A.T. descends slightly. The Mount Clay Loop enters from the left a few feet later, and the A.T. begins to ascend gradually. At mile 12.7, the Westside Trail leads right to Lakes of the Clouds Hut. The A.T. ascends between the edge of the Great Gulf and the Mount Washington Cog Railway.

At mile 13.1, when the Great Gulf Trail descends into the Great Gulf, the A.T. turns right, crosses the cog railway, and continues across the side of Mount Washington. Intersect and turn onto the Trinity Heights Connector Trail, which you follow to the summit of Mount Washington (elevation 6,288 feet) at 13.4 miles.

From here, you take the Tuckerman Ravine Trail for 1.7 miles to Hermit Lake Shelter and Tent site, and another 2.4 miles to Pinkham Notch at NH 16 where you began your hike.

TRAILHEAD DIRECTIONS

Pinkham Notch, the AMC Visitor Center, and the trailhead for the A.T. can be reached by following NH 16 for 8 miles north of Jackson, or for 12 miles south of Gorham.

ZEALAND FALLS, ETHAN POND, AND WEBSTER CLIFFS

MODERATE

25.7 MILES
LOOP

Located along the edges of the Pemigewasset Wilderness, this hike takes you on a moderate ascent to Zealand Falls Hut, where you can enjoy a nice swim at the top of the falls as you gaze out to the mountains in the east. From the falls it is a gradual descent to pretty Ethan Pond, home to both moose and bear. Many have been spotted there so keep an eye out. Tamarack, also called the Eastern Larch, lines the shores of the pond.

The descent from the pond is long and gradual, but get ready for some major huffing and puffing once the hike crosses US 302 and climbs steadily to superb views from Webster Cliffs, Mount Webster, Mount Jackson, and Mount Pierce.

Regulations on camping and fires in the White Mountains change from time to time. Get the latest information from the visitor center at Crawford House, or, to be on the safe side, just plan on camping at the designated campsites. You might also consider treating yourself to a stay in Zealand Fall Hut and/or Mizpah Spring Hut.

If you intend to stay at one of the huts (as opposed to a tent site or shelter), you must make reservations through the Appalachian Mountain Club (AMC). Call (603) 466-2727 or write to Reservations, AMC, P. O. Box 298, Gorham 03581. Fees are inexpensive for tent sites and shelters (close to $10 per person), but hut fees are around $90 per person, which includes lodging, breakfast, and dinner.

The Hike

From the Crawford House parking area, take the Avalon Trail westward to gain about 900 feet in 1.4 miles to the junction with the A-Z Trail, which you then follow. After a bit of a descent and a short, steep climb, most of the route on this pathway has very little change in elevation, so it is a pleasant walk through a predominantly northern hardwood forest. At 5.1 miles, intersect and turn left onto Zealand Trail, passing by attractive Zealand Pond to intersect the A.T. at 5.4 miles. Bear right and make the quick ascent to Zealand Falls Hut at 5.6 miles. The hut is perched dramatically on a rock facing with Zealand Falls right next to it. The view from here is equally dramatic, looking onto the ragged peaks of the southern White Mountains.

When you're ready to leave, take the Trail back to its junction with Zealand Trail and bear right to follow the white blazes of the A.T. (called the Ethan Pond Trail throughout this section), along the gentle grade of an old railroad bed. Keep left at 7.3 miles, when Zeacliff Trail comes in from the right. If you're feeling energetic, you might want to take a short side path to the right to the falls on the Thoreau Falls Trail at 8.1 miles.

Continuing along the A.T./Ethan Pond Trail, keep left as Shoal Pond Trail comes in from the right at 8.6 miles; soon the A.T. leaves the railroad grade, but continues with a gradual descent. At 10.6 miles, it is worthwhile to take the short side pathway to the left to appreciate the serene setting of Ethan Pond and its accompanying campsite. One

mile beyond here, the A.T. bypasses Willey Range Trail coming in from the left and begins a nearly 2,000-foot descent. Along the way it also bypass Kendrum Flume Trail coming in from the left at 14.4 and Arethusa–Ripley Falls Trail going off to the right at 16.0 miles.

Arriving at US 302 at 16.5 miles, cross the road and steeply start to regain the elevation (and more) that you just lost; follow the white blazes of the A.T./Webster Cliff Trail. Eventually, you will come to a viewpoint, the Trail stays along the cliffs, and steadily gains elevation. Cross over the top of Mount Webster at 19.8 miles, bypass Webster-Jackson Trail coming in from the left and, after a series of ups and downs, attain the summit of Mount Jackson where you'll go by another section of the Webster-Jackson Trail at 21.2 miles. There are impressive views from here out across the Presidential Range to Mount Washington.

Going through several alpine meadows, reach Mizpah Spring Hut and Nauman Tent site at 22.9 miles. So as to experience a bit of the terrain above–tree line, continue following the A.T. to the summit of Mount Pierce (4,310 feet above sea level). There is a grand view of the Presidential Range, the sloping expanse of the Dry River drainage system, and of the mountains to the north and west.

Just beyond, at 23.8 miles, the Webster Path comes to an end and you'll now leave white blazes to bear left and descend along Crawford Path. At 24.9 miles, Mizpah Cutoff Trail comes in from left; stay right and continue on a fairly comfortable grade. US 302, Crawford House, and the end of the hike are reached at 25.7 miles.

Trailhead Directions

Trailhead parking is available at Appalachian Mountain Club's Crawford House Hostel and Visitor Center on US 302 about 11 miles north of Bartlett.

FRANCONIA RIDGE AND LONESOME LAKE

This hike begins in Franconia Notch at the junction of US 3 and the A.T. You will hike northward over Franconia Ridge, descend to Franconia Notch via the Old Bridle Path, pick up the Lonesome Lake Trail, and follow it to Lonesome Lake Hut where you will reconnect with the A.T. and hike north to Franconia Notch.

This is a attractive loop hike, taking in both the splendor of Franconia Ridge and the beauty of the Lonesome Lake area. The hike along Franconia Ridge is above–tree line and passes over the summits of Mount Lafayette and Mount Lincoln. Tree line occurs at 4,200 hundred feet; you will hike several miles across the ridge among the krummholz (stunted spruce) and alpine vegetation. Keep to the Trail to avoid damaging these very fragile plants. Franconia Ridge is exposed to sudden and severe storms. Be prepared by bringing along raingear and a warm sweater or coat.

Lonesome Lake is a high mountain tarn on the shoulder of Cannon Mountain. The A.T. follows Cascade Brook, passing its waterfalls and cascades, downstream to Franconia Notch. The Lonesome Lake Trail ascends to Lonesome Lake Hut from Lafayette Campground through the woods along the shoulder of Cannon Mountain.

Franconia Notch—the beginning, middle and end of the hike—features several interesting geological features that can be viewed after your hike. They can all be reached off US 3. The Basin, located 1 mile north of the A.T. crossing on US 3, is a glacial pothole more than 20 feet in diameter; it was carved in granite at the base of a waterfall more than 25,000 years ago. Nearby on US 3 used to be the Old Man of the Mountains, a 40-foot stone profile of a man formed by five ledges of Camon Mountain. It stood more than 1,200 feet above Profile Lake, but broke off and fell from the mountain in 2003. The Flume, also in Franconia Notch, is about a mile south of the Trail crossing off US 3. This natural chasm is 800 feet long with granite walls 60 to 70 feet high, and 12 to 20 feet wide.

If you intend to stay at one of the huts (as opposed to a tent site or shelter), you must make reservations through the Appalachian Mountain Club (AMC). Call (603) 466-2727 or write to Reservations, AMC, P. O. Box 298, Gorham New Hampshire 03581. Tent sites and shelters are close to $10 per person, but the hut fee is around $90 per person, which includes lodging, breakfast, and dinner.

Lodging is also available at Lafayette Campground, which you walk by on this hike. It is operated and maintained by the New Hampshire Division of Parks, and has tent sites, showers, water, a telephone, and some provisions. A fee is charged.

The Hike

From the parking area at US 3 in Franconia Notch, take the mile-long Whitehouse Trail to its junction with the A.T./Liberty Spring Trail. Follow the A.T./Liberty Spring Trail north. In 0.6 mile, reach the junction with the Flume side trail. Continue on the A.T., climbing sharply to Liberty Spring tent site at 3.6 miles. Water is available from the spring located near the Trail at the campsite.

Continue to ascend steeply, and reach Franconia Ridge in another 0.2 mile. The A.T. turns north (left) onto Franconia Ridge Trail, and ascends gradually then steeply over rough ledges. The Franconia Ridge Trail also leads south 0.3 mile to the summit of Mount Liberty. The Osseo Trail starts on top of Mount Liberty and descends south to Kancamagus Highway.

At mile 5.7, you will top Little Haystack Mountain (elevation 4,760 feet). Falling Waters Trail descends from here to Lafayette Campground on US 3, but you will reach the same campground later by way of the Old Bridle Path.

Continue on the A.T., which is now above–tree line. At mile 6.4, you will reach the summit of Mount Lincoln (elevation 5,089 feet), and at mile 6.8, a minor peak. Ascend steeply up the rocky cone of Mount Lafayette (elevation 5,249 feet), and reach the summit and the intersection with the Greenleaf Trail at mile 7.4.

Close to the remains of the summit house foundation, take the Greenleaf Trail to the left, descend a short distance to a spring, and hike to Greenleaf Hut at 8.5 miles. At Greenleaf Hut, pick up the Old Bridle Path and hike 2.5 miles down the mountain to Lafayette Campground at US 3.

Lonesome Lake Trail leaves Lafayette Campground at US 3 and travels just over 1 mile to Around-Lonesome-Lake Trail. This 0.3-mile trail leads around the northern shore of Lonesome Lake to Lonesome Lake Hut and the Appalachian Trail.

In 0.1 mile, you will reach the junction of the A.T./Fishin' Jimmy Trail with the A.T./Cascade Brook Trail. You want to follow the A.T. as it runs concurrently downstream with the Cascade Brook Trail along Cascade Brook, the outlet stream of Lonesome Lake.

At mile 13.2, the Kinsman Pond Trail enters from the right. Continue downstream along the A.T. for 0.5 mile and cross the wooden bridge over Cascade Brook. Shortly thereafter, reach the Basin–Cascade Trail, which heads left to The Basin on US 3.

Continue on the A.T./Cascade Brook Trail, cross over Whitehouse Brook, and go under both lanes of US 3 at 15.2 miles, where you will soon turn right onto the Whitehouse Trail to retrace your steps back to the beginning trailhead at 16.2 miles.

Trailhead Directions

The Appalachian Trail crossing at US 3 is 5.8 miles north of North Woodstock. However, you must park south of the A.T. at the Whitehouse Trail and Flume Center (also called the New Hampshire State Park Flume Complex) and hike 1 mile north to the Trail crossing via the Whitehouse Trail.

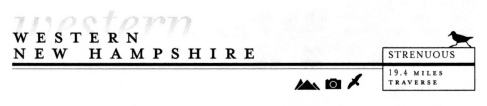

WESTERN
NEW HAMPSHIRE

STRENUOUS

19.4 MILES
TRAVERSE

During this overnight hike, you might be lucky enough to spot a Peregrine Falcon. A reintroduction program at Holts Ledge has been successful, and falcons have been nesting below the ledge since 1987. There might be signs posted to keep hikers away from the nesting area. Human intrusion could jeopardize the rearing of the young, so please don't be tempted to venture beyond the signs.

On this traverse, there are a few steep climbs and descents, but a number of places offer spectacular views of the surrounding countryside. You can hike from either direction, but we suggest starting at New Hampshire 25A and traveling south. It gets the toughest climbs out of the way early and leaves the easier sections for the second day. If you prefer to tackle the tougher climbs and descents on the second day, you will want to hike north from Goose Pond Road. Smarts Mountain Shelter and Tent site makes a nice location to camp, and it divides the outing into two hikes of roughly equal length.

The Hike

From the trailhead at NH 25A, hike south on the A.T. and begin ascending Mount Cube. At mile 1.8, cross Brackett Brook and continue climbing. In another 1.5 miles,

reach the col between the summits of North and South Cube. A short side trail leads to the summit of North Cube, which—of the two peaks—affords the better view of the White Mountains. Continue on the A.T. and reach the summit of South Cube (elevation 2,911 feet) in 0.2 mile. From the open summit, you can look ahead to your next climb, Smarts Mountain.

Follow the A.T. down from Mount Cube for 1.4 miles, then cross a small stream just before the 0.3-mile side trail to Hexacuba Shelter. Water for the shelter is available from the creek at the junction of the side trail with the A.T. Continue following the A.T. south, crossing two brooks and a couple of old logging roads in the next 1.4 miles. The second brook—Jacobs' Brook—at mile 6.4, is at the base of the climb up Smarts Mountain. The Trail climbs steadily for 3.8 miles to the summit of Smarts (elevation 3,240 feet).

The old Firewarden's Cabin is maintained as a hiker shelter, and there is a tent platform on the summit as well. Water is available from a spring 0.1 mile away on a blue-blazed side trail. The view from the fire tower is outstanding, but the view from the privy is one of the best on the mountain.

From the summit of Smarts Mountain, descend on the A.T. and reach the junction with the Smarts Mountain Ranger Trail in

0.5 mile. Continue following the A.T. and cross the rocky Lambert Ridge, where there are fine views from several points on the ridge, and reach the parking lot on the Lyme-Dorchester Road 3.8 miles south of Smarts Mountain.

Continue following the A.T. across Lyme-Dorchester Road, then immediately make a turn to the right. Watch for other turns. Cross Lyme-Dorchester Road at 16 miles and begin the moderate climb to Holts Ledge. From the road, hike 0.9 mile to the 0.2-mile side trail for Trapper John Shelter. Water is available from a creek near the shelter. Reach the high point of the Trail on Holts Ledge 0.5 mile past the shelter side trail. A 0.1-mile side trail leads to the top of the Dartmouth College Skiway and the viewpoint at Holts Ledge. Follow the A.T. down from the Ledge for 2 miles and reach Goose Pond Road.

Trailhead Directions

The A.T. crosses NH 25A 4.3 miles west of Wentworth. Limited parking is available. The southern end of this hike is on Goose Pond Road, 3.3 miles east of New Hampshire 10. Goose Pond Road turns left off New Hampshire 10 about 3 miles south of Lyme.

From the Connecticut River at the Vermont–New Hampshire border, the Appalachian Trail passes from east to west, crosses through hardwood forests and climbs over hills dotted with pastures and fields. This area features cleared hills, pastures, ravines, steep hills, and patches of timber. Stone walls, cellar holes, and other remnants of the farms that once dominated this area can still be seen. The area is now reverting to forest.

Vermont
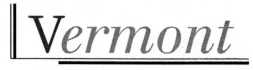

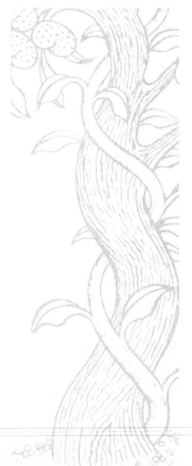

The A.T. joins the Long Trail near Sherburne Pass, where it heads more than 100 miles south to the Vermont–Massachusetts border. The A.T climbs the slopes of Pico and Killington Peaks of the Coolidge Range, part of the Green Mountains, and reaches its highest point in Vermont just below Killington Peak (elevation 4,235 feet). After passing over the Coolidge Range, it descends and crosses Clarendon Gorge on a suspension bridge. In the Green Mountains, the A.T. traverses the main ridge, passes mountain ponds, and crosses several peaks, including Peru Peak, Spruce Peak, and Stratton Mountain. The latter is said to be the birthplace of the A.T. From Stratton, the Trail continues to Glastenbury Mountain before descending to Vermont 9 near Bennington. It follows a ridge for 14 miles until it meets the Vermont–Massachusetts border.

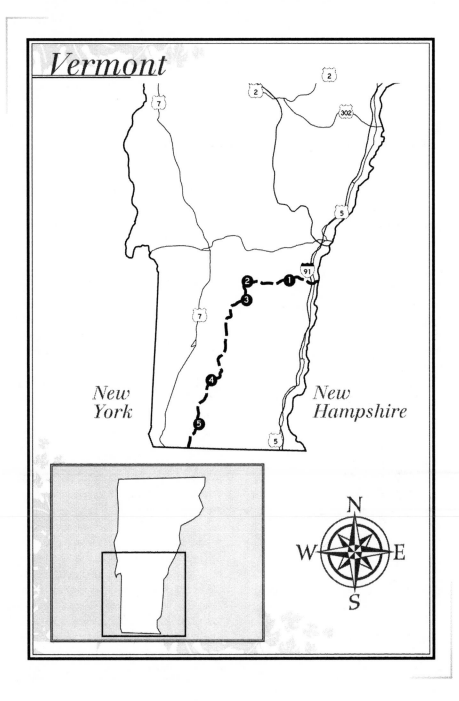

Vermont

7

2

2

302

7

5

91

2

3

1

7

4

5

New York

New Hampshire

5

N
W E
S

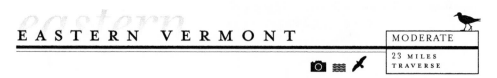
On this hike, you will be traversing an intermountain range section as the A.T. makes its way from the White Mountains of New Hampshire to the Green Mountains of Vermont. The elevations along this hike are not that extreme, between 1,500 and 2,500 feet above sea level, but there are plenty of ups and downs along the way.

You will enjoy fine views at Lakota Lake Lookout, pass the beautiful Kent Pond, and cross a portion of Gifford Woods State Park. The state park is along a major migratory bird flyway, and bird watchers flock to the park in the spring and fall to see the varied birds that use it as a rest area during their migration. The park also boasts a virgin grove of forest made up largely of sugar maples.

There is an optional side trip near the end of this hike. The Deer Leap Trail climbs to the top of Deer Leap Cliffs and affords outstanding views of Sherburne Pass and its surrounding peaks.

The Hike

From the trailhead on Barnard Gulf Road, follow the A.T. south. At mile 1.1, enjoy good views from an open ridge top (Mount Ascutney is to the south). At mile 2.2 and mile 3.1, cross old roadbeds. At mile 3.7, reach the 0.2-mile side trail to Wintturi Shelter. Water is available from a small spring near the shelter.

The Trail then ascends more steeply as you continue to climb over and down Sawyer Hill. At mile 5, the A.T. turns right onto King Cabin Road. In another 0.2 mile, the Trail turns off the road—watch for the turn.

At mile 6.1, reach the junction with the Lookout Spur Trail. This side trail ascends 0.2 mile to the Lookout, a private, locked cabin that has an observation deck available to hikers. It overlooks one of the best views on the hike. Continue following the A.T. for 1.7 miles to reach the Lakota Lake Lookout. There are good views of the lake as well as the surrounding countryside, while the White Mountains appear in the distance.

For the next several miles, you will be following a ridge with occasional knobs to climb. Cross Lost Creek and Chateauguay Road at mile 8.9, and pass a small pond at mile 10.9. The end of the ridge is descended by way of switchbacks. At mile 13.3, you will reach the short side trail to Stony Brook Shelter immediately before the first of two stream crossings.

Cross Stony Brook Road in 0.1 mile and begin climbing steadily. Reach the top of a ridge and cross a shoulder of Quimby Mountain on the way to the highest point of the hike, an unnamed mountain (elevation 2,640 feet) at mile 15.1. Descend steeply on switchbacks to a ridge and cross under power lines, where there are good views from the power line right-of-way. Climb to another unnamed point and descend gradually and hike to a viewpoint from an old logging road at mile 16.8.

At mile 17.6, cross gravel River Road and follow Thundering Brook Road across the Ottauquechee River. The A.T. turns off the road, climbs gradually over a hill, and rejoins the road again in 0.4 mile. The Mountain Meadows Lodge is to your left just after you pass the dam for Kent Pond. As you follow the shoreline, you will pass a swimming area and cross a few small creeks.

At mile 19.9, the A.T. joins Vermont 100 for a short distance before turning off the highway into Gifford Woods State Park. Shelters and tent sites are available for rent. The A.T. winds its way through the park, passing the caretaker's house, showers, camping area, and more. Beyond the park, the A.T. ascends, sometimes steeply, and reaches the junction with the Sherburne Pass Trail, a former route of the A.T., which descends 0.5 mile to US 4 in Sherburne Pass.

Continue on the A.T. to the western intersection with the Deer Leep Trail. This pathway climbs sharply 0.3 mile to the top of Deer Leap Cliffs for an outstanding view of Sherburne Pass and surrounding peaks before continuing for another 1 mile to rejoin the A.T. further south. If you decide to take this side route, you will only add about 0.5 mile to the hike as the Deer Leap Trail comes to its eastern junction with the A.T. at mile 21.9. From that intersection, it is only 0.1 mile to the "Maine Junction." The A.T. and the Long Trail go south and share the same pathway to the Massachusetts border. The L.T. also heads north to the Canadian border. Continue following the A.T. and descend to US 4 at mile 23.

TRAILHEAD DIRECTIONS

The Trail crosses Vermont 12 at Barnard Gulf Road, 4.4 miles north of Woodstock. There is a parking area at the road crossing. For the trailhead at the southern end of the hike, the A.T. crosses Vermont 4, 8.6 miles east of Rutland.

PICO PEAK

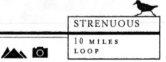

STRENUOUS

10 MILES
LOOP

In the 1990s, the Appalachian Trail was relocated away from ski resort development on and near Pico Peak and removed from its traverse through Sherburne Pass. However, the old route remains open as the blue-blazed Sherburne Pass Trail and makes for a great loop hike of 10 miles when combined with the new section of the A.T. The outing could be accomplished as a day hike. Yet, there are so many good places to linger and enjoy views and the scenery beside the Trail that it should be done as an overnighter.

You have the choice of staying in one of three shelters, or of treating yourself to a night in the historic Inn at Long Trail. For reservations, call (800) 325-2540.

THE HIKE

From the trailhead on US 4, follow the A.T. south. Cross a stream at 1.8 miles, and ascend gradually via switchbacks. Pass the 0.1 mile side trail to Churchill Scott Shelter at 1.9 miles. The water source is a seep located a short distance south of the shelter. Be aware that it should not be counted on in times of dry weather. Continuing on the A.T., pass Mendon Lookout at 2.2 miles. The Trail ascends through a spruce-fir forest with the dogwood-like blossom of bunchberries spreading across the forest floor from May into July.

At 3.8 miles, leave the white blazes of the A.T. and turn left onto one of its former routes, now known as the blue-blazed Sherburne Pass Trail. Come to Pico Camp, a cabin for overnight stays, at 4.3 miles. Water is available from a spring a short distance beyond the shelter. Behind the camp, climb the steep blue-blazed Pico Link Trail 0.4 mile to the summit of Pico Peak for views across the mountains and down onto several ski trails.

Return to Sherburne Pass Trail and turn left to descend to US 4 in Sherburne Pass at 7.6 miles. Cross the highway (use caution as cars speed by), pass the Inn at Long Trail, and continue to follow the Sherbune Pass Trail as it rises to meet the A.T. at 8.1 miles.

Turn left onto the A.T. to the western intersection with the Deer Leep Trail. This pathway climbs sharply 0.3 mile to the top of Deer Leap Cliffs for an outstanding view of Sherburne Pass and surrounding peaks before continuing for another 1 mile to rejoin the A.T. further south. If you decide to take this side route, you will only add about 0.5 mile to the hike as the Deer Leap Trail comes to its eastern junction with the A.T. at 8.9 miles. From that intersection, it is only 0.1 mile to the "Maine Junction." The A.T. and the L.T. go south and share the same pathway to the Massachusetts border. (The L.T. also heads north, 0.4 mile to the Tucker–Johnson Shelter and more than 160 miles to the Canadian border.)

Continue following the A.T. and descend to US 4 at mile 10.

TRAILHEAD DIRECTIONS

The Trail crosses US 4, 8.6 miles east of Rutland.

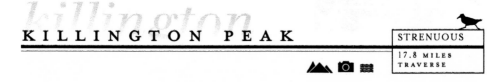

KILLINGTON PEAK

STRENUOUS

17.8 MILES
TRAVERSE

This hike traverses the Coolidge Range of the Green Mountains and reaches the highest elevations along the Appalachian Trail in Vermont. A short side trail leads to Killington Peak (elevation 4,235 feet). It is from the summit of Killington that the state was christened "verd mont" or "green mountains" in 1763. From the top of Killington, you can see the Green Mountain Range of Vermont—from Glastenbury Mountain in the south to Mount Mansfield in the north. There are also views of the White Mountains of New Hampshire, the Taconics and Adirondacks of New York, and, on clear days, you can make out landforms in Massachusetts, Maine, and even Canada.

The evergreen forests and dense hardwoods along this section provide for an especially spectacular traverse in the fall. In the lower half of this section, you will find yourself descending into foothills, and winding through pastures, fields, open woods, and second-growth conifers.

THE HIKE

From the trailhead on US 4, follow the A.T. south. Cross a stream at 1.8 miles, and ascend gradually via switchbacks. Pass the 0.1 mile side trail to Churchill Scott Shelter at 1.9 miles. The water source is a seep located a short distance south of the shelter. Be aware that it should not be counted on in times of dry weather. Continue on the A.T., and pass Mendon Lookout at 2.2 miles. The Trail ascends through a spruce-fir forest with the dogwood-like blossom of bunchberries spreading across the forest floor from May into July.

Keep to the right as you pass by the Sherburne Pass Trail (a former route of the A.T.) at 3.8 miles. Pass the Bucklin Trail coming in from the right at 6.2 miles; a short distance later pass Cooper Lodge (elevation 3,900 feet), where there is a spring 100 feet south of the cabin. At 6.3 miles, take the 0.2 mile side trail that leads steeply to the summit of Killington Peak (elevation 4,235 feet), which is above–tree line and is the second highest mountain in Vermont. There is a very expensive snack bar on the summit as well as a chairlift (open Memorial Day through Labor Day). However, you will also be rewarded with one of the most spectacular views in Vermont.

Back on the A.T., continue south through a saddle between Killington and Little Killington. At 8.4 miles, the Shrewsbury Peak Trail heads left. Keep right on the A.T., descend, and cross a number of old logging roads and streams to arrive at Governor

Clement Shelter at 10.9 miles. Water is available from the stream across the road to the east. Continue across the clearing, into the woods, and turn right onto a woods road.

A short distance later, the Trail turns left off the road, crosses Robinson Brook, ascends, and then turns left along the western bank of the brook. The Trail continues with minor elevation changes. Reach an old road at mile 11.7, turn sharply left, cross Sargent Brook, turn right, and follow the brook downstream.

In 0.6 mile, you will cross Upper Cold River Road and continue to descend along Sargent Brook. In another 0.7 mile, cross Gould Brook and descend along its left bank. At 13.8 miles, turn right on Cold River Road (Lower Road), cross a concrete bridge, turn left into the woods, and follow the western bank of Northam Brook uphill. In 0.3 mile, leave the brook, cross a field, and soon turn left onto Keiffer Road.

Within a few feet, turn right off the road; and ascend along a stone wall. Reach the crest of the ridge at 15.2 miles and pass the unreliable Hermit Spring 0.3 mile later.

Cross the unpaved Lottery Road at 15.9 miles. Be sure to close the farm gates as you ascend a pasture, climbing to a grove of sugar maples. At mile 16.3, reach the airport beacon atop Beacon Hill (elevation 1,760 feet). The Trail drops steeply and crosses a brook in 0.5 mile to reach Crown Point Military Road—built during the French and Indian War. The Clarendon Shelter is 0.1 mile away, via a trail to the left. The A.T. continues south, crosses a town road, climbs gradually to a rock promontory, and descends through a steep gorge.

Cross a couple of stiles, and come to Vermont 103 at 17.8 miles. Clarendon Gorge is on the other side of VT 103 and is spanned by the Mill River Suspension Bridge. There is good swimming here, but refrain from diving off the rocks.

For the northern trailhead, the Trail crosses US 4, 8.6 miles east of Rutland. For the southern trailhead, the A.T. crossing at VT 103 is 2.4 miles east of US 7, 7.3 miles south of Rutland, and 6.2 miles west of East Wallingford.

LITTLE ROCK POND TO CLARENDON GORGE

MODERATE

14.8 MILES
TRAVERSE

This is one of the best hikes on the A.T. in Vermont. The gentle climb from the road to Little Rock Pond is a great way to get out and stretch your legs. The initial portion of trail runs alongside Little Black Brook, and many small waterfalls and pools are visible from the Trail.

The clear, cold water of the pond reflects Green Mountain rising above it on the opposite shore. It is a popular day hike to the pond, particularly in the fall. The foliage around the pond is breathtaking at its peak. If you want to have any solitude, try to do this hike during the week or leave the trailhead by 10 a.m. to beat the crowds. However, the number of hikers thins out considerably once you hike beyond the pond. The climb of White Rocks Mountain is long, but ascends at a relatively gradual rate.

The expansive view from White Rocks Cliff is reached by a short side trail from the A.T. Directly below the wide quartzite cliffs, a talus slope bordered by a spruce forest directs your view into the deep valley carved by the erosive waters of Otter Creek. The small town of Wallingford is to the northwest along the banks of the stream. The Adirondacks of New York are on the western horizon.

After several ups and downs and miles to the north along the A.T., you will reach Clarendon Gorge. Here you may swim in the narrow gorge where you can sit in potholes created by Mill River and let the swirling waters relax you with nature's own whirlpool. You could also sunbathe on the flat rocks situated in the shallower water above the gorge.

THE HIKE

From the trailhead at the parking lot on USFS 10 (Danby-Landgrove Road), hike north on the A.T. and pass by the short side trail to Lula Tye Shelter at 1.7 miles. Reach the southern end of Little Rock Pond at 1.9 miles. From here, the Little Rock Pond Loop Trail skirts the west side of the pond. The A.T. stays on the eastern side, soon passing the Little Rock Pond Tenting Area and a spring, before coming to the northern end of the pond at 2.2 miles. The Green Mountain and Homer Stone Brook Trails come in from the left. Stay right and pass by the Little Rock Pond Shelter side trail at 2.4 miles.

Cross Homer Stone Brook at 3.3 miles and traverse the long ascent of White Rocks Mountain. At 6.3 miles, turn left onto the

White Rocks Cliff Trail. A steep, rocky descent of 0.2 mile brings you to the cliffs, where you might have the opportunity to watch a dozen or more turkey vultures soar upon the thermals rising from the valley floor.

Return to the A.T. and continue north, where at 7.1 miles you will pass by the Greenwall Spur Trail, which leads 0.3 mile to Greenwall Shelter. Continue on the A.T. to cross Bully Brook and pass by Keewayding Trail coming in from the left at 7.7 miles. Cross Sugar Hill Road at 8.4 miles, step across the bridge over Roaring Brook, and reach Vermont 140 at 8.5 miles.

Cross the road diagonally to the right and ascend to a side trail at 9.5 miles, which goes left for 100 feet to a view of White Rocks. Continue on the A.T., ascend and then descend to the side trail at 12.1 miles, which leads 200 feet to Minerva Hinchey Shelter.

Controlled burns, used to keep lands open for wildlife, provide a view to the west of New York's Taconic Range at 12.7 miles, while Airport Lookout also enables you to gaze onto the Taconics at 14 miles. The hike is almost over when you reach Mill River passing through Clarendon Gorge at 14.7 miles. So, take a break by following the pathway down to the water (please do not create new trails) for a swim and sunbath. When done, follow the A.T. across the bridge to the end of the hike on Vermont 103 at 14.8 miles.

TRAILHEAD DIRECTIONS

For the southern trailhead, the A.T. crosses Danby-Landgrove Road (USFS 10) 3.5 miles east of US 7 in Danby. Parking for the northern trailhead is on VT 103, 2.4 miles east of its intersection with US 7 north of Clarendon.

STRATTON MOUNTAIN AND LYE BROOK WILDERNESS LOOP

STRENUOUS

23.2 MILES
LOOP

This is actually a figure-eight hike that will take you through some of the best the Green Mountains have to offer. The hike uses the A.T. and L.T., the Lye Brook Trail, the Branch Pond Trail, and the Stratton Pond Trail to wind you through the Vermont wilderness. Stratton Mountain is topped with a fire tower offering a commanding view of the Green Mountains and surrounding Vermont countryside. You will also hike to Stratton and Bourn Ponds and pass through the Lye Brook Wilderness.

There are several shelters and tent sites along this hike, supplying numerous options for breaking up this outstanding hike. Stratton Pond is the one of the busiest spots on the Long Trail. A caretaker is on duty in peak season and fees are charged for staying in the shelter.

Although rated moderate, the hike up and back down Stratton Mountain is definitely strenuous. Don't despair; the rest of the hike is much easier.

The Hike

From the trailhead on Arlington–Wardsboro Road (locally known as Kelly Stand Road), hike north on the A.T., which on this section shares the same pathway with the L.T. You will gradually begin ascending, and in 1.4 miles, you will cross a dirt road. The ascent becomes more strenuous as you climb Stratton Mountain. At mile 3.1, pass a small spring on the uphill side of the Trail.

At mile 3.8, reach the wooded summit of Stratton Mountain (elevation 3,936 feet). It is worth the effort to climb to the top of the fire tower and take in the tremendous view. Stratton and Bourn Ponds can be seen to the west far below. Mount Equinox, the highest peak in the Taconic Range, is also to the west. Glastenbury Mountain is to the southwest, Mount Pisgah to the south, Mount Monadnock to the southeast, and Ascutney Mountain to the northeast.

Follow the A.T. off the summit and descend steeply for the first mile, then more gradually. Reach an old road 2 miles past the summit of Stratton. At mile 6.9, the Stratton Pond Trail goes left 0.1 mile to Stratton Pond Campsite Shelter and another 3.6 miles to Arlington–West Wordsboro Road. Continue on the A.T. for 0.1 mile and make a left turn onto blue-blazed Lye Brook Trail, as it runs along the southern shore of Stratton Pond. Passing by the junction with the North Shore Trail, you will soon cross over Winhall River (where you enter the 14,300-acre Lye Brook Wilderness) and come to South Bourn Pond Shelter at 9.5 miles. From the South Bourn Pond Shelter, follow the Branch Pond Trail north for 0.5 mile and pass a short side trail leading to the North Bourn Tenting Area, which offers a privy and a couple of tent platforms. Near the platforms, there is a good view of Stratton Mountain rising above the pond.

From the camping area, soon cross Bourn Brook and follow the Trail to the William B. Douglas Shelter 3.8 miles from the South Bourn Shelter. Water is available from a spring along the Trail before you reach the shelter. From the Douglas Shelter, hike 0.5 mile to the junction with the A.T. Turn back hard to your right and follow the A.T. south for 2.8 miles to a bridge over the Winhall River. Cross the bridge, and climb along the side of an unnamed ridge before descending to the northeastern corner of Stratton Pond and the junction with the North Shore Trail in 1.8 miles.

Continue to follow the A.T. south and keep right when the Lye Brook Trail comes in from the left in 0.1 mile. In another 0.1 mile, turn right onto the blue-blazed Stratton Pond Trail, soon coming to the Stratton Pond Campsite Shelter. This was the route of the A.T. until a 1989 relocation over Stratton Mountain. With little elevation change, the Stratton Pond Trail continues 3.6 miles to Arlington–West Wardsboro Road. When you reach the road, turn left and walk the 0.9 mile back to the parking area at the trailhead.

Trailhead Directions

The A.T. crosses Arlington-West Wardsboro Road (locally known as Kelley Stand Road) 13.2 miles east of US 7 at Arlington.

The Appalachian Trail enters Massachusetts 4 miles north of a road crossing (Massachusetts 2 in North Adams), descending along the rocky ridge of East Mountain. From North Adams, the Trail continues up Prospect Mountain Ridge and over Mount Williams and Mount Fitch to the summit of Mount Greylock, the highest point in Massachusetts (elevation 3,491 feet).

Massachusetts

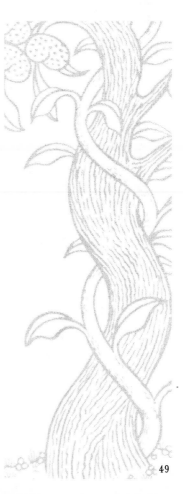

From Mount Greylock, the A.T. descends to Cheshire, heads to Dalton, and climbs the Berkshire Hills. The Trail traverses High Top and passes by Finerty Pond before entering October Mountain State Forest. After crossing US 20 at Greenwater Pond, the A.T. continues to Upper Goose Pond and descends into the Tyringham Valley. The A.T. then enters Beartown State Forest, skirting Benedict Pond.

From here, the Trail heads southwest into East Mountain State Forest, crosses over Warner and June Mountains, and descends to the Housatonic River. The last miles of the A.T. in Massachusetts cross the valley to the Taconic Range, climb Mount Everett and Mount Race, pass beautiful Bear Rock Falls, and descend to the Connecticut border in Sages Ravine.

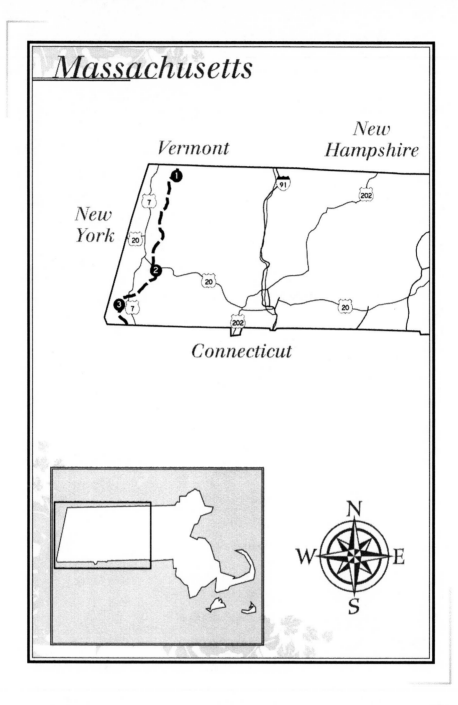

Massachusetts

New Hampshire

Vermont

New York

Connecticut

MOUNT GREYLOCK LOOP

MODERATE

10.9 MILES
LOOP

This short overnight loop uses the Hopper Trail, the Money Brook Trail, and the A.T. to form a hike through the Mount Greylock State Reservation, which is situated on 11,000 acres. The highlight is the summit of Mount Greylock (the highest point in Massachusetts), where the first observation tower in the nation to charge admission is located. The summit now boasts the Massachusetts War Memorial (no fee), a stone structure on the site of the former observation tower.

The summit also houses Bascom Lodge, which offers private and bunk room accommodations (with shared baths), snack bar, and family style dinners. Call (413) 743-1591 for reservations and more information.

Beyond the summit, the hike passes Wilbur Clearing, named for Jeremiah Wilbur who used to pasture his animals on the 1,600 acres around this old corral—now a small grassy area in the middle of a red spruce grove.

Camping is not permitted in the North Adams–Mount Williams Reservoir watershed on the northern side of Mount Greylock.

THE HIKE

The hike begins at Hopper Road where both the Hopper Trail and the Money Brook Trail begin. From the farm gate on the road leading between two pastures, follow the road for 0.1 mile to the second farm gate with stone walls on both sides.

In another 0.2 mile, you will reach the junction with the Money Brook Trail, which leads downhill to a brook. The Hopper Trail heads into an overgrown pasture. After taking the right fork onto the Hopper Trail through the pasture, enter the woods at 0.5 mile, and begin a steady climb through an open hardwood forest.

At mile 1.4, a side trail heads left, downhill, to the Money Brook Trail. In another 0.1 mile, you will reach several springs that come out of the side of the hill and cross the Trail. This is the only available water on the Hopper Trail.

In another 0.8 mile, after a steady, and at times quite steep ascent, the Trail levels off in a red spruce grove and passes site 16 of the Sperry Campground at Sperry Road. The Hopper Trail follows Sperry Road for 0.1 mile before heading left back into the woods opposite the campground's contact station. The Trail here is both steep and wet.

In 0.1 mile, you will see the remains of an old CCC log dam and spring house below a cliff, and a small waterfall to the right. In another 0.1 mile, the Hopper Trail turns left sharply as the Deer Hill Trail (the old Greylock Stage Coach Road) enters from the right. For the next 0.5 mile, you will follow this road up Mount Greylock. Reach the junction with the Overlook Trail to the left and hike another 0.1 mile to the junction with Rockwell Road.

Walk 0.2 mile through the woods to reach Rockwell Road at its junction with the A.T. and the Cheshire Harbor Trail. Turn left onto the A.T. and skirt the south side of an old water-supply pond for 0.2 mile before reaching the junction of Notch Road, Summit Road, and Rockwell Road. You will hike through woods of stunted spruce and fir before emerging into a clearing next to a television tower.

Attain the summit of Mount Greylock (elevation 3,491 feet) at 4.1 miles. Climb the monument tower for a view of Bascom Lodge, the Berkshire Hills to the south, and the Green Mountains of Vermont to the north. After continuing north toward the end of the parking lot, the A.T. descends and crosses Summit Road, eventually leveling off on the ridgeline where Thunderbolt and Bellows Pipe Trails head east. The A.T. continues over an usual outcropping of milky quartz on the round, tree-covered top of Mount Fitch at mile 5.4.

In 0.8 mile, a side trail leads 0.3 mile to Notch Road. The A.T. continues to ascend steadily, passing the blue blazes and granite marker that indicate the western boundary of the North Adams Watershed. At mile 6.4, the Trail passes by a register atop Mount Williams. Cross Notch Road at mile 7.3 (near the day-use parking area), and hike 0.1 mile to the junction of the Money Brook Trail. The 0.3 mile side trail to Wilbur Clearing Lean-to is also located at this junction.

Leaving the A.T. and heading through the red spruce grove on the Money Brook Trail, you will soon pass a spring, and in 0.2 mile, the Wilbur Clearing Lean-to will appear on the right. In another 0.3 mile, a short-cut trail to Notch Road comes in from the left as you pass through a beech and northern hardwood forest.

After a steep sidehill descent, you will come to a hairpin turn in the Trail, where there is a side trail to the left to Money Brook Falls. Descending through a hemlock grove, you will cross Money Brook for the first time at mile 8.3. Continue to descend gradually along a shelf parallel to the brook, and reach the junction of the Mount Prospect Trail in another 0.8 mile. The Mount Prospect Trail ascends steeply from the brook to the right.

Stay on the Money Brook Trail, and in 0.1 mile, you will cross Money Brook again, and then one of its tributaries. Continue downstream along Money Brook for 0.4 mile to the side trail short cut to the Hopper Trail on your left. Take a sharp left across a tributary of Money Brook, and find a large pool at the junction of the two main tributaries that form Hopper Brook.

The Trail follows an old logging road for 0.5 mile, and crosses Hopper Brook. In another 0.2 mile, you will reach a fence next to a brookside pasture. Follow the farm road uphill and reach the junction with the Hopper Trail in 0.2 mile. In another 0.2 mile, you will once again pass the gate, which has stone walls, to reach your waiting automobile.

TRAILHEAD DIRECTIONS

Access Hopper Road off Massachusetts 43 in Williamstown The trailhead is at the end of Hopper Road, where there is a designated parking area near the Haley Farm.

FINERTY POND TO BENEDICT POND

MODERATE

📷 〰 🏠

30.1 MILES
TRAVERSE

From the scenic Finerty Pond at the northern end of this section, past the wide expanse of Upper Goose Pond, to the glacial Benedict Pond near the southern end, you will pass through the beautiful Massachusetts woods and near the picturesque town of Tyringham. This section also crosses Webster Road, the site of a two-school community that thrived in the early 1800s. It was home to Widow Sweets, a self-taught bonesetter and local legend.

South of Tyringham, you pass the site of the former Tyringham Shaker Community (1792-1875). All that remains are cellar holes and wide stone walls. This section leads through farm and hay fields before it reaches the Beartown State Forest. The Trail also passes through a steep valley before climbing to The Ledges with views of Mount Everett and the Catskills.

While the terrain crossed on this hike is fairly moderate with only a few short, steep uphills, it can be a long hike for some people to accomplish in two days. You could turn it into a three-day outing of hikes of almost equal lengths by staying in the cabin or tent site at Upper Goose Pond the first night and the Shaker Campsite the second night.

Camping is only permitted at designated sites throughout this hike.

THE HIKE

The A.T. follows a dirt service road to the south from Pittsfield Road, but leaves it in 0.1 mile to soon enter October Mountain State Forest. Containing more than 14,000 acres, it is Massachusett's largest state forest. Cross unpaved Dirt Branch Road at 1.5 miles. The large, 12-person October Mountain Lean-to is located along a short trail that intersects the A.T. at 2.2 miles.

It may get a bit noisy at 3.3 miles, where you cross over the Gorilla Trail, a motorcycle-ATV route. Rise over Bald Mountain (no views) at 3.8 miles and walk along County Road for 300 feet before reentering the woods at 4 miles. Cross several streams around 5 miles and an old logging road (now used by ATVs) at 5.5 miles. Begin walking beside Finerty Pond at 6.2 miles. This lovely body of water, which provides excellent swimming opportunities, was once a swamp. In the 1930s, the Civilian Conservation Corps dammed its outlet stream to create a water reservoir for Lee.

Leave the pond and rise slightly to the overgrown summit of Walling Mountain at 7.1 miles and pass over the top of Beckett Mountain (again, no views) at 8.1 miles. Cross Tyne Road at 8.6 miles, and US 20 (Jacob's Ladder Highway) at 9.4 miles.

Following the A.T. south from US 20, you will cross a stream on a high bridge at a historic mill site beside the outlet of Greenwater Pond. At 9.8 miles, cross the Massachusetts Turnpike (I-90) on twin bridges, enter the woods, and climb steeply up a rough trail.

Within the next 0.6 mile, you will cross two intermittent brooks and reach the top of the ridge, where there is a register box and an overlook of the Upper Goose Pond Natural Area. At 11 miles, the A.T. takes a sharp left turn at its junction with the side trail to the Upper Goose Pond Cabin, 0.5 mile away. A caretaker is on duty at the cabin, and there is a fee for both tent sites or bunkroom space.

Continue along the A.T. for 0.3 mile and pass an old chimney and a plaque marking the site of the former Mohhekennuck fishing and hunting club. Hike for 0.5 mile along the shore of Upper Goose Pond, purchased by the National Park Service for the A.T. corridor. Upper Goose Pond is one of the more outstanding features along the A.T. in Massachusetts. Walking beside this pretty New England pond, you will discover the reason for its name—it is the nesting site of many Canada Geese.

Cross the inlet of the pond. Soon, you will pass a spring to the right and soon thereafter leave this protected natural area as the Trail heads away from the pond to climb steeply, and then descend almost as steeply. At mile 13.5, reach the outlet of a beaver marsh on a long bridge constructed of telephone poles. The Trail continues through ferns and ground pine with the marsh to the left. In 0.1 mile, you will parallel a stone wall and then cross a small brook.

There is a house visible to the left as the Trail passes through a mostly level pine forest. Cross the dirt Goose Pond Road (Tyringham Road) in another 0.1 mile. The Trail gently ascends and descends through a hemlock grove before reaching a side trail that leads to a view of a pond.

At mile 16.1, after crossing a swiftly flowing inlet, you will cross Webster Road. For the next 0.2 mile, you will pass over cobbles before reaching a plateau and overgrown fields. Hike 1.7 miles to Main Road, which leads right 0.9 mile to the town of Tyringham.

After crossing Main Road, you will pass over Hop Brook on a bridge. Use bog bridges to follow fencing and hedgerows around wet fields. You will also pass over a gas line swath and reach crisscrossing brooks in a hemlock grove at mile 18.

Hike another 0.3 mile and cross Jerusalem Road. Enter the Tyringham Cobble Reservation. Here, open fields are managed to help out the wildlife; no camping or fires are permitted. Climb up Cobble Hill and reach the high point at mile 19.4, where there is a good view of the Tyringham Valley. Following the Trail through the field, you soon enter a pine forest.

In another 0.6 mile, you will begin to switchback down through a hemlock grove, and leave the Reservation lands. Hike 0.3 mile and enter another hay field. Follow the edge of the field for 0.1 mile.

Cross a hedgerow and another small brook, and you will enter another hay field. Follow the edge of this field, too, and enter the woods in 0.1 mile. After passing over a cleared gas-pipeline crossing at mile 20.6, and another hay field with good views of the valley to the north, you will enter the woods to the left. Step over a small dirt berm and cross two small streams. Pass by the Shaker Campsite at mile 20.9. Nearby is a waterfall and the remains of the former Shaker community.

Begin to switchback uphill to Fernside Road at 21.2 miles, where there is a spring a short distance east. Cross the road and follow the A.T. up the steep bank, and soon reach a logging road that switchbacks up the ridge.

In 0.5 mile, you will reach the top of a white pine knoll and begin to descend. Turn sharply at a boulder gulch along cliffs covered with fern. You might notice that the temperature is cooler here. At mile 22, you will reach a view of the Tyringham Valley, and at mile 22.7, three stone walls to the right that mark the boundary of the Beartown State Forest.

In another mile, the A.T. turns sharply west into a hemlock grove to bypass a swamp. After crossing a west-flowing brook between the swamps, the A.T. reaches another corner of the Beartown State Forest and turns south again.

At mile 24.4, the Trail crosses Beartown Mountain Road at a culvert for a brook that supplies the beaver ponds. In 0.1 mile, after skirting a planted Norway spruce grove, the A.T. crosses a motorcycle trail and ascends. After 0.5 mile, the A.T. joins a blue-blazed trail for 600 feet on top of the ridge. Here also is the 0.25-mile side trail to the Mount Wilcox North Shelter. It sleeps eight to ten, but the water source is uncertain during the dry season.

After 0.6 mile, the Trail skirts the east side of Beaver Pond and crosses its outlet, and in another 0.5 mile, reaches the top of a plateau with a view to the south. At mile 26.8, locate the Mount Wilcox South Shelter a short distance to the left of the Trail. Water is available from a spring on a side trail. Another spring is a short distance south on the A.T. The Trail then crosses a woods road and two small brooks before climbing steeply.

At mile 27.5, the A.T. skirts the edge of the Ledges. Enjoy views of East and Warner Mountains, Mount Everett, and the Catskills. After 0.2 mile, the Trail crosses the outlet of a swamp and beaver dam, turns left, and descends steeply down the slope of a ravine.

After turning left on an abandoned road 0.3 mile later, cross a bridge, turn right off the road, and skirt the eastern shore of Benedict Pond at 28.1 miles. A short distance later, you will cross a state forest road that leads right to a picnic area, telephone, and outhouse.

Hike 0.4 mile, ascend slightly, turn right and follow a woods road as it passes an old charcoal pit. At mile 29.1, cross about 100 yards of swamp over bog bridges and rocks steps, then turn southeast away from the corner of a pasture. After a gentle ascent and descent of an overgrown pasture (another 0.5 mile), the Trail crosses an intermittent stream in a steep gully. Leave the gullies for higher ground, and pass through an area damaged by a tornado in 1995. Reach Massachusetts 23 at 30.1 miles.

TRAILHEAD DIRECTIONS

Roadside parking is available for the northern trailhead on Pittsfield Road, 8 miles southeast of Pittsfield and 5 miles northwest of Beckett. The Trail crossing at the southern end of the hike is on MA 23, 4 miles east of Great Barrington.

JUG END, MOUNT EVERETT, AND SAGES RAVINE

STRENUOUS

16.5 MILES
TRAVERSE

Some of the best hiking the A.T. has to offer in Massachusetts and Connecticut is packed into this one overnight hike. You will pass several magnificent viewpoints, but the highlight of this hike is perhaps at one of its lowest points, Sages Ravine.

There are several particularly good tent sites that break up the trip nicely into two sections. One camp lies near the banks of Sages Ravine Brook, which tumbles through the lush growth of the ravine in a seemingly unending series of beautiful small waterfalls and pools of clear, cold water. Another, Bear Rock Falls Campsite, has more than 50 acres surrounding it. The land was donated to the Appalachian Trail Conference in memory of three hikers—Susan Hanson, who died in a 1990 plane crash, and Geoffrey Hood and Molly LaRue, who were murdered during a southbound thru-hike of the A.T. in 1990. A granite marker has been placed at the bottom of Bear Rock Falls, a cascade of more than 300 feet, to commemorate the hikers.

THE HIKE

From Jug End Road, hike south on the A.T. and begin a moderate ascent. In 0.25 mile, the Trail ascends more sharply, and steadily climbs up Jug End. The summit is reached at mile 1.1, where you are treated to a spectacular view, which takes in much of the Berkshire Hills to the north—including Mount Greylock.

Cross two unnamed peaks on your way to Mount Bushnell (elevation 1,834 feet) at 2.3 miles, and pass by the Elbow Trail at 2.8 miles. At mile 3.4 is the short side trail to small Glen Brook Lean-to. In 0.1 pass the side trail to Hemlocks Lean-to. The water source for both shelters is from the stream at this trail junction.

From the side trail junction, hike 0.3 mile to the Guilder Pond Loop, which goes around Massachusetts' second highest pond (elevation 2,042 feet). The loop trail for the pond uses a portion of the A.T. to complete the loop. Stay on the A.T. and reach the Guilder Pond Picnic Area in 0.1 mile and continue following the white-blazed A.T. Climb the north slope of Mount Everett and reach the summit at mile 4.6.

From the summit of Mount Everett (elevation 2,602 feet), there is a commanding 360-degree view of the Taconic and Berkshire Ranges, the Housatonic River Valley, and the distant Catskills. The pitch pines around the summit are said to be dwarfed by poor soil, not by altitude. Look at the rock surface beneath your feet, and you will see scrapes and pits that were created as glaciers slid along the top of this mountain during the last Ice Age.

The steep and rocky 0.7-mile descent off Mount Everett brings you to a sag between Mount Everett and Mount Race, and the junction with the Race Brook Trail. Continue following the A.T. for 1.1 miles, climbing to the summit of Mount Race (elevation 2,365 feet). The Trail follows a rocky ledge along the side of the mountain, offering fine views of the Housatonic River Valley to the east.

At mile 8.1, cross Bear Rock Stream. On your left is the camping area at the top of Bear Rock Falls. The campsite has established fire rings and a privy. The sunrise from the rock outcrop in the camping area can be magnificent; just be careful, as injurious falls have occurred here.

One mile beyond the campsite, begin the short descent into Sages Ravine. At mile 9.5, cross Sages Ravine Brook on a footbridge. There are designated campsites and a privy at 10.1 miles. A caretaker is in residence during the summer, but no fee is charged. No fires permitted.

At mile 10.2, reach the junction with the Paradise Lane Trail. Continue following the A.T. for a steep and rocky ascent of Bear Mountain. At 10.9 miles, the Trail reaches the summit of Bear Mountain (elevation 2,316 feet). This is not, as once believed, the highest point in Connecticut (though a monument from 1885 says otherwise). The state's high point (elevation 2,380 feet) is on the south slope peak of nearby Mount Frissell that is in Massachusetts.

Views from the ruins of the stone tower include the Twins Lakes, Canaan Mountain, and Haystack Mountain to the east; across the Berkshires to Mount Greylock in the north; and the New York Catskill Mountains to the west. The Housatonic Valley stretches out to the south.

From Bear Mountain, hike along an old charcoal road that the A.T. follows briefly. At mile 11.8, reach Riga Junction, where you will pass by the Undermountain Trail. Hike 0.5 mile to walk past the short blue-blazed side trail to Brassie Brook Campsite and Lean-to. Water is available from the small stream on the A.T. just before the side

trail. Hike another 0.6 mile to Ball Brook, where the Ball Brook Campsite is located just before you cross the brook. At 13.5 miles is a short side trail to Riga Lean-to and Camping Area (water is from a spring near the shelter), which boasts a fine view of the valley below. The mountain you are walking upon drops precipitously down a cliff face revealing a broad valley of small towns and farm fields that is speckled by the waters of Washenee and Washining Lakes, better know as the Twin Lakes.

The junction with the Bald Peak Trail, which leads to private property, is 0.2 mile beyond the Riga Lean-to side trail. Hike another 0.4 mile to the north lookout of Lions Head, with views of Bear Mountain and Mount Greylock to the north. This is also the point with the northern intersection of the blue-blazed Bypass Trail. Reach Lions Head at 14.2 miles (elevation 1,738 feet), with views south and east to Salisbury, Lakeville, and Wetauwanchu Mountain. Twin Lakes is visible to the northeast. The south junction with the Bypass Trail is 0.1 mile beyond. In another 0.1 mile, pass the junction with the Lions Head Trail and continue following the A.T. along a moderate, then gradual 2.3-mile descent to the Plateau Campsite. Descend another 0.2 mile to the trailhead on Connecticut 41.

TRAILHEAD DIRECTIONS

From MA 41, 6 miles north of the state line of Massachusetts–Connecticut, turn left on Curtiss Road. Curtiss Road becomes Jug End Road and reaches the trailhead in 1.5 miles. There is adequate parking at the trailhead.

The southern trailhead is a parking lot on CT 41 (Undermountain Road), 0.75 mile north of its junction with US 44 in Salisbury, Connecticut.

THE APPALACHIAN TRAIL TRAVERSES 52 MILES OF CON-
NECTICUT. FROM THE STATE LINE OF MASSACHUSETTS,
THE A.T. CLIMBS BEAR MOUNTAIN AS IT ENTERS CON-
NECTICUT. THE TRAIL FOLLOWS THE TACONIC RANGE
TO ITS SOUTHERN END AT LIONS HEAD WHERE THERE IS
AN OUTSTANDING PANORAMIC VIEW. THE A.T. THEN
CROSSES A FEW MOUNTAINS AND FOLLOWS ALONG THE
HOUSATONIC RIVER.

Connecticut

THE MOUNTAINS IN CONNECTICUT ARE ALL LESS
THAN 2,400 FEET IN ELEVATION, YET THERE ARE
MANY FINE VIEWPOINTS IN THIS SECTION OF THE A.T.
THE HIGH POINTS—LIONS HEAD, RAND'S VIEW,
HANG GLIDER VIEW, AND OTHERS—OFFER COM-
MANDING VIEWS OF THE COUNTRYSIDE.

IN FALLS VILLAGE, THE A.T. FOLLOWS A PORTION OF
THE RIVER TRAIL, ONE OF THE FIRST SECTIONS OF
THE TRAIL'S 2,100 MILES TO BECOME WHEELCHAIR
ACCESSIBLE. THE A.T. CROSSES INTO AND OUT OF
NEW YORK ON THE SIDE OF SCHAGHTICOKE MOUN-
TAIN, AND THEN PASSES INTO NEW YORK AT HOYT
ROAD, 7 MILES FARTHER.

CAMPING IS PERMITTED ONLY AT DESIGNATED SITES
IN CONNECTICUT. FIRES ARE PROHIBITED ANYWHERE
ALONG THE TRAIL'S TRAVERSE OF THE STATE.

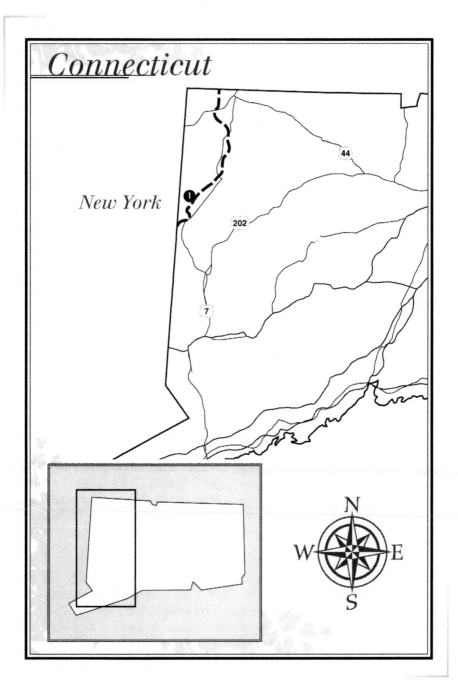

1. Housatonic River to Ten Mile Hill

HOUSATONIC RIVER TO TEN MILE HILL

MODERATE

23.1 MILES
TRAVERSE

This traverse takes you along an Appalachian Trail relocation that opened in 1988, removing the A.T. from Cornwall. After climbing Silver Hill and passing the largest big-tooth aspen tree in Connecticut (just south of Swift's Bridge), the Trail reaches River Road and follows the Housatonic River for close to 5 miles—one of the longest river walks on the entire A.T. Along the way, the Trail passes through a grove of red pine that is dying of blight. The trees were planted as an experiment in the early 1930s.

The section from St. Johns Ledges to Connecticut 341 is located in the township of Kent. This area was Native American land for thousands of years, but by 1752, only eighteen out of the approximately 100 families inhabiting the area remained and most of the land had been sold off. Some of the archaeological sites along the Housatonic River date back more than 9,000 years.

Near Indian Rocks, the A.T. passes through the Schaghticoke Indian Reservation, crosses into New York for a short distance, and returns to Connecticut to run close to Bulls Bridge over the Housatonic River. It is one of the few remaining covered bridges in Connecticut and one of only two that still carries traffic. It is worth it to take the few steps over to see it, and if the water is not running high, the river just below the bridge may entice you into a swim.

After a short diversion over a small rise, the A.T. returns to the Housatonic River, where you can gaze upon its numerous small cascades and waterfalls and enjoy the shade of the many hemlock trees. Another swim may be in order as the Trail crosses Ten Mile River before ascending to Ten Mile Mountain for the final view of the journey.

THE HIKE

Walk westward on Connecticut 4 for 0.5 mile and turn left onto the A.T. to follow it to the south. At 0.6 mile, climb very steeply to the height of the land, and enjoy good views. Reach the side trail to Silver Hill Campsite, the site of the former Silver Hill Shelter at 1.4 miles. The shelter burned to the ground in 1991 because of a faulty fireplace; a waterpump, covered cooking area, and privy are still usable. Cross Dawn Hill Road at mile 2, and River Road at 2.2 miles. There is a piped spring a few feet to the left. The A.T. continues along the road, and just beyond the spring, you will find the site of Swift's Bridge. Three different bridges have crossed the river here, but all were destroyed; the last one by a flood in 1936. The A.T. leaves the road, goes down an embankment and picks up the old River Road, with the river on one side and hay fields on the other. The fields are locally known as Liner Farm. In another 2 miles, you will cross Stony Brook, where camping is permitted in the designated sites on the south side of the stream.

At 4.6 miles, cross Stewart Hollow Brook and reach the side trail to the Stewart Hollow Shelter. Water is available from the brook, which flows out of a pasture, so make sure you treat the water. From the shelter side trail, hike through the red pine plantation. Even though most of the trees are now dead, the walk through the grove is still eerily beautiful. Members of the Appalachian Mountain Club—Connecticut Chapter harvested some of the dead and dying trees to build four of the A.T. shelters in Connecticut, including the Ten Mile River Lean-to you will pass later in this hike.

At mile 5.9, pass the gate at the site of the old North Kent Bridge, which was destroyed by a flood in 1936. The A.T. once crossed the Housatonic River here. In another 0.4 mile, cross a stream, and shortly reach the base of St. Johns Ledges at 6.9 miles. Entering the woods, you will ascend 90 stone steps installed by a trail crew from the Appalachian Mountain Club. You may also see rock climbers on the nearby cliffs. Hike 0.5 mile to the top of the ledges and find wonderful views of the Housatonic River Valley and the town of Kent. Hike another 0.7 mile to the top of Caleb's Peak (elevation 1,160 feet). The outcropping along the ledges affords good views to the south. From here, the A.T. turns left and descends through the woods.

At mile 8.6, enjoy more good views from a ledge outcropping, and 0.2 mile later, cross Skiff Mountain Road. At mile 8.9, cross Choggam Brook, which is often dry in late summer. Hike 1.9 miles to another ledge that provides views of Kent and the Housatonic River Valley. At mile 11, pass the old A.T., which leads straight ahead to Numeral Rock. The old A.T. can be used as a bypass when Macedonia Brook floods; otherwise continue another 0.5 mile and cross

Macedonia Brook on a log bridge. Walk through a pasture, cross Connecticut 341 at 11.6 miles, and ascend through the woods.

At mile 11.9, a side trail leads right to water and the Mount Algo Lean-to. Continue along the A.T. and reach the height of the land at mile 12.5. Cross Thayer Brook at mile 12.9. After Thayer Brook, ascend a rocky route to the high point of Schaghticoke Mountain at mile 13.4. From here, the Trail follows ledges that offer good views to the south.

At 14.8 miles, descend into Rattlesnake Den, a ravine with large hemlocks and tumbled boulders. After crossing a brook, you will ascend gradually, passing by the side trail to the Schaghticoke Mountain Campsite, with water and a privy.

In another 0.3 mile, descend into Dry Gulch, a rocky ravine, and climb out of it, steeply. From here, you will climb along the eastern slope of Schaghticoke Mountain and reach Indian Rocks at mile 15.4. This overlook has views to the east of the Housatonic River Valley. Around this area, the A.T. passes through the Schaghticoke Indian Reservation on a narrow corridor of trail lands. This is the only Native American property the A.T. courses through on its route from Maine to Georgia.

A marker identifies where you cross into New York at 15.8 miles, but there may be no sign to let you know you walk back into Connecticut as you descend switchbacks a short distance later. Turn left onto Shaghticoke Road at 18.7 miles and follow it for 0.3 mile to turn right and ascend into the woods. Covered Bulls Bridge and great swimming in the Housatonic River are just a few steps away by continuing to follow the road to the left.

Go over a rise with less than 70 feet of elevation gain and come back to the Housatonic River at 19.5 miles. The Trail follows an old road on a high bank above the river, giving you the opportunity to enjoy the stream and maybe catch a great blue heron trolling the shallow waters in search of a meal. Walk through a break in a stone wall at mile 20, a reminder of the days when this land was used for agricultural purposes. A power line right-of-way opens up a view of Ten Mile Hill to the south.

Cross Ten Mile River on the Ned Anderson Memorial Bridge at 20.1 miles. Anderson was a Connecticut farmer who built and maintained the original route of the A.T through the state for two decades. If you did not stop to take a swim at Bulls Bridge, you might want to consider one here. Afterwards, walk by the Ten Mile River Camping Area (privy available) and begin to ascend. Pass the side trail to Ten Mile River Lean-to at 20.3 miles and the blue-blazed John Herrick Trail 1.1 miles later.

Reach the summit of Ten Mile Hill at 21.3 miles and take the short side trail to the view of the Housatonic Valley. Continuing on the A.T., cross Connecticut 55 at 22.4 miles, rise and descend across a low ridge, and come to the end of the hike when you reach Hoyt Road at 23.1 miles.

Trailhead Directions

For the northern trailhead, the A.T. crosses CT 4, 0.9 west of Cornwall Bridge. However, you must park 0.5 mile to the east, where US 7 joins CT 4. For the southern trailhead, drive New York 55 east from Wingdale, New York, for 3.3 miles, and turn right onto Hoyt Road. The A.T. and parking area are reached in another 0.25 mile.

The 92 miles of the A.T. in New York travel from Schaghticoke Mountain on the Connecticut line to the Kittatinny Range in New Jersey, passing through Fahnestock and Harriman–Bear Mountain State Parks. Just south of the Bear Mountain Bridge, the A.T. reaches its lowest point at the Trailside Zoo in Bear Mountain Park (elevation 124 feet). Hikers are no longer charged a toll for walking across the bridge.

New York

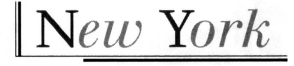

Part of the Trail a short distance south of the Bear Mountain Bridge was the first section of the A.T. to be built. It was cleared in 1923 by a group from the New York–New Jersey Trail Conference. That group still maintains the Trail in both states.

New York City's skyline can be seen on a clear day from several points along the A.T. in New York, including West Mountain Shelter and Mombasha High Point. After passing through Harriman–Bear Mountain State Parks, the A.T. travels west, then south, leaving New York near Prospect Rock.

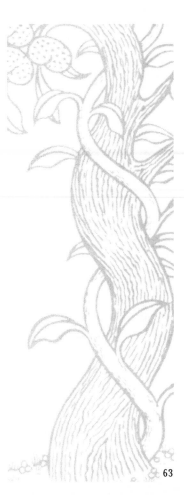

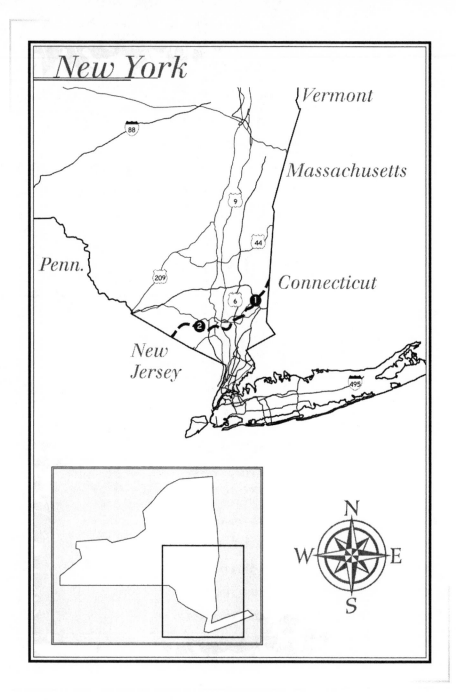

New York

Vermont

Massachusetts

Penn.

Connecticut

New Jersey

SHENANDOAH MOUNTAIN TO
BEAR MOUNTAIN BRIDGE

A t the start of this two-day traverse, you will cross Shenandoah Mountain, which affords good views from the summit. You will also pass a particularly nice view of Canopus Lake. As you follow an old narrow-gauge railroad bed, you will pass through an area that saw much activity during the Revolutionary War.

Near the end of the hike, you will follow the ridge as it descends steeply down Anthony's Nose on the way to the Bear Mountain Bridge. There are several theories on when and why the ridge was named Anthony's Nose. The Appalachian Trail Guide to New York–New Jersey lists three probable explanations: 1) In 1525, a Portuguese sailor, Estevan Gomez, named the ridge for the Hudson River, which he called Rio St. Antonio; 2) Diedrich Knickerbocker's History of New York claims it was for Anthony Corlear, also known as Anthony the Trumpeter; and 3) Some believe the ridge was dedicated to Revolutionary War General "Mad" Anthony Wayne, who led the march that successfully wrested nearby Stony Point from British control. The Thru-Hiker's Handbook lists a fourth explanation for the ridge's name. According to that book, the ridge was called Anthony's Nose after the navigator on Henry Hudson's ship, the Half Moon.

After crossing the Bear Mountain Bridge, you will pass through the Trailside Museum and Zoo. The original idea for the Appalachian Trail, as put forth by Benton

MacKaye in the 1920s, included a number of such exhibits along the route.

THE HIKE

From Horntown Road at Ralph's Peak Hikers' Cabin, follow the A.T. south. In 1 mile, cross over a high point on Shenandoah Mountain, descend 0.2 mile to the level of the ridge, then begin the often steep ascent of Shenandoah Mountain. At mile 1.8, pass under power lines in a utility right-of-way, and at mile 2.4, cross Long Hill Road. Continue climbing and reach the summit of Shenandoah Mountain (elevation 1,282) at mile 2.8. The mostly open summit has fine views to the east.

Descend 0.4 mile from the summit to an old woods road, and follow along the roadbed for the next 0.7 mile. In another 0.7 mile, reach the junction with a short side trail that leads to a viewpoint. At mile 4.7, reach an overlook with an outstanding view of Canopus Lake below. An unmarked trail leads east around the lake and about 0.5 mile to the state park campground. Descend from the viewpoint to a ridge paralleling Canopus Lake, which can be seen through the trees to the left of the Trail.

At mile 6.9, reach New York 301, turn left, and follow the white blazes along the road. Cross the road in 0.1 mile and walk into a grove of hemlocks. For the next 0.7 mile, the Trail follows an old railway bed used to haul ore down from Sunk Mine. At mile 7.7, the A.T. turns to the left off of the railroad bed, and in 0.2 mile, reaches the junction with the Three Lakes Trail. Continue following the A.T. and climb to a ridge top in 0.6 mile. In another 0.6 mile, the Trail briefly joins Sunk Mine Road, then turns left into the woods, climbs to a high point on a ridge, and descends.

Pass by Catfish Loop Trail at mile 10.5, and cross Dennytown Road at mile 10.7. Water is available from a pump beside the stone building about 200 feet east along the road. After reentering the woods, the A.T. briefly shares the trailway with the blue-blazed Three Lakes Trail. At mile 11.9, pass by the southern junction with the red-blazed Catfish Loop Trail. Continue following the A.T., cross a stream, and step over South Highland Road at mile 13.4. One mile after this, cross Canopus Hill Road and enter the woods. Hike 0.7 mile to the top of Canopus Hill to enjoy limited views.

After a short, steep descent off of Canopus Hill, the Trail climbs once more before descending to the intersection of Chapman Road and Albany Post Road (mile 16.1). After crossing the roads and reentering the woods, the A.T. passes through a marshy area on bog bridges and then climbs to the top of Denning Hill (elevation 960 feet). You can see New York City to the east on a clear day. This is the northernmost place the city is visible from the A.T. In another 0.3 mile, reach the junction with a 0.1-mile side trail leading to a memorable view of the Hudson River.

The Trail climbs over Little Fort Hill, and at mile 18.1, a side trail leads to Graymoor Monastery, where there are views to the east. From the Monastery side trail, hike 0.7 mile to cross Old West Point Road. In another 0.4 mile, cross Old Highland Turnpike, then cross a swampy area on bog bridges before reaching US 9 at mile 19.4.

After crossing US 9 at its junction with New York 403, continue following the A.T.

south, and walk through a pasture on bog bridges. Pass by the intersection with the yellow-blazed Carriage Connector Trail, and the junction with the blue-blazed Osborn Loop Trail in another 0.5 mile. At 20.5 miles is a junction with a short side trail leading to an excellent vista. From this viewpoint, you can see the Hudson River below. The Bear Mountain Bridge is visible to the left.

A number of marked and unmarked trails join the A.T. in this area; be sure to follow the well-blazed A.T. At mile 22.8, reach South Mountain Pass, a dirt road the Trail briefly follows before turning left on another dirt road. Follow the second dirt road for 0.2 mile before turning off and reaching the side trail to Hemlock Springs Campsite. Water is available from the spring.

From the side trail to the campsite, hike 0.8 mile to another dirt road. At mile 24 is the blue-blazed trail to the summit of Anthony's Nose. It is well worth the time and effort to take the 1.2 mile round-trip journey to the summit. In a sweeping vista from south to north, your gaze can take in Iona Island jutting out into the river, Bear Mountain rising high from the opposite bank with Hessian Lake in front of it, and the houses and roadways of Fort Montgomery. The skyline of New York City may be seen about 50 miles to the south on clear days.

Continue on the A.T. and descend rather steeply for 0.5 mile to New York 91. Turn left and follow the highway for 0.2, before turning right and crossing Bear Mountain Bridge. Hikers are not charged a toll as they once were.

Turn left into the Trailside Museum and Zoo at mile 25.2. The zoo closes at 4:30 p.m.; you must walk around it if you arrive later. The lowest spot on the entire Appalachian Trail—elevation 124 feet—is in the zoo. Pass through the zoo and hike 0.8 mile to the southern trailhead at the Bear Mountain Inn.

The first exit south of I-84 on the Taconic State Parkway is Miller Hill Road. Turn right onto Miller Hill Road and then take your first left onto Horntown Road. Park about 0.1 mile from Miller Hill Road, where the A.T. crosses Horntown Road. At this point you will see a former private residence, now maintained as the Ralph's Peak Hikers' Cabin. It is not named for a nearby mountain but for a dirt pile dubbed Ralph's Peak that once graced the lawn. The dirt pile is gone, but the name stuck. Adequate parking is available at the house.

The southern trailhead is at the Bear Mountain Inn in Bear Mountain State Park on New York 9W near the Bear Mountain Bridge and the Palisades Parkway. A fee may be charged.

HARRIMAN STATE PARK

MODERATE

17.5 MILES
TRAVERSE

On this overnight hike, you will cross New York's Harriman State Park. The park was conceived by Edward Harriman who made his fortune in railroads and dreamed of creating a park in this area. After his death, his widow helped to make the dream a reality. She donated 10,000 acres to the state for use as a park with the condition that New York abandon plans to build a prison on lands it had acquired around Bear Mountain. The state agreed, and Bear Mountain and Harriman Parks were born. The parks are also the site of the first section of pathway built (in 1923) specifically for the A.T.

As you cross Bear, West, Black, Letterrock, Fingerboard, Island Pond, and Green Pond Mountains, you will find many fine views along the way. This hike takes you past the ruins of Civil War–era Greenwood Mine and within sight of Lake Tiorati. The Trail through Harriman exhibits the Trail builders' sense of humor (if not ingenuity) as you wiggle your way through the tight-fitting section of trail known as the "Lemon Squeezer."

During this hike description, you will read about a number of other trails that meet, cross, or share the footpath with the A.T. For more information about those trails and other hiking opportunities in the area, read *Harriman Trails: A Guide and History* by the New York–New Jersey Trail Conference.

Throughout this hike, camping is permitted only at shelters.

THE HIKE

From the trailhead near the Bear Mountain Inn, hike south on the A.T. on the paved path along the shore of Hessian Lake, and turn left at the playground. The A.T. shares this section of trailway with the yellow-blazed Suffern-Bear Mountain Trail. As you begin climbing, cross under the ski jump in 0.2 mile and briefly join a gravel road. After leaving the gravel road, hike to where the Suffern–Bear Mountain Trail continues ahead and the A.T. turns right. From this trail junction, continue on the A.T. and hike 0.4 mile to the paved Perkins Drive. Enjoy the views of the Hudson River and Bear Mountain Bridge.

At mile 1.3, use the steps as you continue climbing Bear Mountain. Cross Scenic Drive a couple of times, and at mile 1.8, reach the summit of Bear Mountain (elevation 1,305 feet), where there is a sweeping view to the east of the countryside and the New York City skyline. There is also a stone observation tower, water fountain, and rest rooms.

From the summit, continue following the paved road for 0.1 mile, leave the road, descend, and reach Perkins Drive at 2.4 miles. Follow Perkins Drive for 0.5 mile and then reenter the woods. In another 0.5 mile, cross Seven Lakes Drive and follow an old woods road. At mile 3.5, reach the junction with the red-blazed Fawn Trail. Continue on the A.T. and begin sharply ascending West Mountain. From the Fawn Trail junction, hike 0.5 mile to a point offering fine views to the east. In another 0.1 mile, the A.T. joins the blue-blazed Timp–Torne Trail. The two trails share the same footpath for the next 0.7 mile. As you climb West Mountain, there are several views from the rocky ledges.

At mile 5, the Timp–Torne Trail turns off to the left. West Mountain Shelter is 0.6 mile down the Timp–Torne Trail. There is no water available at the shelter. However, as a consolation, you can see the skyline of New York City from the shelter, and if there is an event, the lights of the Meadowlands in New Jersey can be seen at night.

From the junction of the Timp–Torne Trail (to the left), hike 0.5 mile to Beechy Bottom Road, a bicycle path. In 0.4 mile, reach the junction with the red-on-white-blazed Ramapo-Dunderberg Trail, which shares the trailway with the A.T. for several miles. Cross the Palisades Interstate Parkway at 6 miles. Be particularly careful when making this road crossing; the traffic often goes faster than the speed limit.

From the Parkway, hike 0.3 mile to the junction of the 1779 Trail. Continue following the A.T. and climb, often steeply, for 0.4 mile to the south side of Black Mountain. Enjoy views from the open rock ledges. In 0.4 mile, reach a vista of Silvermine Lake below, then continue descending for 0.1 mile to a cross-country ski trail.

Begin climbing Letterrock Mountain. After crossing an unnamed knob on the ridge, descend to William Brien Shelter at mile 8.1. Water is available from a well on a short side trail. This well is sometimes dry and should not be depended on.

Beyond the shelter, continue climbing Letterrock Mountain and reach the summit (elevation 1,195) in 0.3 mile. Descend 0.5 mile and cross a bridge over a boggy section of trail in the gap between Letterrock and Goshen Mountains. The red-on-white-blazed Ramapo-Dunderberg Trail takes its leave of the A.T., which rises along the side of Goshen Mountain. In 1.2 miles, cross Seven Lakes Drive at an angle, and in another 0.2 mile, cross a bridge over a stream and begin to climb the ridge.

Hike 0.8 mile to a rock outcrop with a fine view of Lake Tiorati. You will briefly follow and cross several old woods roads before descending to Arden Valley Road at mile 12.3. (From this road crossing, it is 0.25 mile to the left to Tiorati Circle where there is a bathhouse, rest rooms, water fountains, and a picnic area. You may want to pick up your water there; it is treated and the side trip is shorter than the 0.5 mile from

Fingerboard Shelter to its water source—Lake Tiorati.)

Continuing on the A.T., cross Arden Valley Road and once again join up with the red-on-white-blazed Ramapo-Dunderberg Trail. (The two trails will share the same footpath for the next 1.2 miles.) In 0.1 mile, pass a water tank and ascend. Reach the summit of Fingerboard Mountain (elevation 1,328 feet) in another 0.4 mile. There is an old stone fireplace on the summit. Descend from the peak and then climb gradually again to the junction with the blue-blazed Hurst Trail that is 0.5 mile beyond Fingerboard Mountain or mile 13.4. You can see Fingerboard Shelter about 100 yards down the Hurst Trail. After passing the Hurst Trail, hike 0.1 mile to where the Ramapo-Dunderberg Trail goes straight and the A.T. turns right. Continue following the A.T. and descend sharply. In 0.5 mile, the Trail follows Surebridge Mine Road and passes close to a water-filled pit. This was the site of the Greenwood Mine, a Civil War–era iron mine. In another 0.1 mile, the Trail crosses Surebridge Brook and climbs for 0.3 mile to a high point on Surebridge Mountain before descending for 0.3 mile to cross an intermittent creek.

At mile 14.9, reach the junction with the blue-blazed Long Path. Continue south on the A.T. and begin the 0.3-mile climb of Island Pond Mountain. On the summit (elevation 1,303 feet), the A.T. joins the red-on-white-blazed Arden–Surebridge Trail. The two trails share the same footpath for the next 0.2 mile as they descend and pass through the Lemon Squeezer. Take the bypass trail if you don't want to follow the blazes down the steep descent and through the narrow passage between the boulders of the Lemon Squeezer. At the bottom of the Lemon Squeezer, the Arden–Surebridge Trail turns left and the A.T. turns right. Follow the A.T. as it winds its way to an old woods road. Turn right and follow the road for 300 feet, crossing an inlet of Island Pond. Turn left off the road and climb to a viewpoint over Island Pond at mile 16. Descend and cross an outlet of Island Pond on a wooden bridge in another 0.1 mile. This outlet is partially channeled into a stone spillway, made of cut stones. This spillway was constructed by the CCC in 1934, as a part of a plan to dam the pond, and thereby enlarge it. However, the work was never completed and the pond remains in its natural state.

After crossing the bridge, climb, and in 300 feet, cross a gravel road which provides access for anglers to Island Pond. Continue following the A.T., cross dirt Island Pond Road, and begin climbing the eastern slope of Green Pond Mountain. After reaching the summit at mile 17.3, descend to the Old Arden Road, which once connected the Arden Estate with the town of Tuxedo. Turn right and follow the road for 0.1 mile to turn left onto paved Arden Valley Road. In another 0.1 mile you will turn into the Elk Pen Parking Area to reach your shuttled car and the end of the hike.

TRAILHEAD DIRECTIONS

The northern trailhead at the Bear Mountain Inn in Bear Mountain State Park is on New York 9W near the Bear Mountain Bridge and the Palisades Parkway. A fee may be charged. The southern trailhead is at the Elk Pen Parking Area on Arden Valley Road, 0.25 mile east of New York 17. Arden Valley Road meets NY 17, 0.75 mile south of the town of Arden.

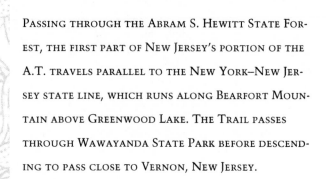

Passing through the Abram S. Hewitt State Forest, the first part of New Jersey's portion of the A.T. travels parallel to the New York–New Jersey state line, which runs along Bearfort Mountain above Greenwood Lake. The Trail passes through Wawayanda State Park before descending to pass close to Vernon, New Jersey.

New Jersey

Crossing the Vernon Valley, a former glacial lake, the Trail crosses Pochuck Creek and attendant swamplands to ascend Pochuck Mountain and descend to the Wallkill Valley. The A.T. continues to High Point State Park after passing close to Unionville, New York. This section of the Trail is characterized by rolling farmland, pastures, fields, and open woods.

Although the A.T. does not actually reach the High Point's summit, there is a short side trail to it. From High Point State Park, the A.T. follows Kittatinny Ridge to Stokes State Forest.

From Stokes State Forest, the Trail continues along Kittatinny Ridge through Worthington State Forest to the Delaware Water Gap National Recreation Area.

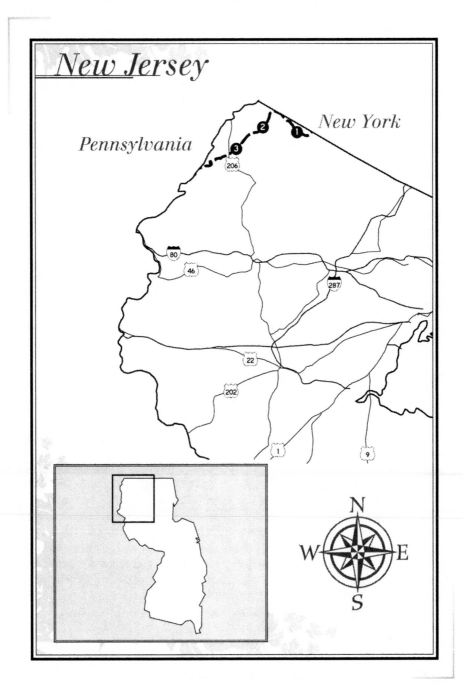

New Jersey

Pennsylvania

New York

1. THE POCHUCK CROSSING AND
   WALLKILL VALLEY
2. KITTATINNY MOUNTAINS

3. DELAWARE WATER GAP AND
   KITTATINNY MOUNTAINS

THE POCHUCK CROSSING
AND WALLKILL VALLEY

MODERATE

11.8 MILES
TRAVERSE

The lowlands of New Jersey are often overlooked as a hiking destination because they don't provide any spectacular mountain views. That may be, but the Trail through here presents an opportunity that is missing in the mountainous areas. You will get the chance to walk close to small residential communities, beside picturesque agricultural lands dotted by grazing cattle, and along the dikes of a former sod farm that is now the protected land of the Wallkill River National Wildlife Refuge, the only national wildlife refuge on the entire Appalachian Trail. You will be hiking through open country a good percentage of the time, so there will be long views across the lowlands to the mountains rising both east and the west.

The swamps and bogs of the lowlands can be a bird-watcher's paradise. According to a list compiled by the U.S. Fish and Wildlife Service, close to 200 species can be seen here. You may have the opportunity to observe herons, egrets, vultures, hawks, plovers, owls, woodpeckers, vireos, thrushes, warblers, finches, sparrows, and more.

As if all of this is not enough, the A.T. also makes use of an engineering marvel. It took 24 years of discussions, planning, and hard work amongst a coalition of many organizations and hundreds of volunteers to enable you to cross what was once known as

the "Pochuck Quagmire." A boardwalk, completed in 2002 and nearly a mile in length with a 100-foot suspension bridge in the middle of it, allows you to cross the fields, swamps, and marshes of Pochuck Creek without getting your feet wet. In dry weather, the creek is not much more than a trickle. In wet weather, it easily overflows its channel, flooding the land and turning it into a half-mile wide lake.

Wheelchair accessible, the boardwalk takes hikers into a land populated by cardinal flowers, goldenrod, thistle, cattails, marsh hawks, black bears, and limestone rock formations rising dozens of feet above the flood plain. The open views from the boardwalk include Pochuck Mountain to the west and Wawayanda Mountain to the east.

The walking is relatively easy, with just one long, gradual rise to the top of Pochuck Mountain. This outing receives a moderate rating only because of its length.

Oh, yeah. One last thing. Do be aware that it can be very hot and buggy during the summer. Consider doing the hike at some other time of year.

THE HIKE

Follow the A.T south and pass through a livestock pasture on bog bridges. At 0.2 mile, use stiles over fences on both sides of the crossing of the New York, Susquehanna, and Western Railway railroad tracks, before walking through more fields. A bridge enables you to cross Wawayanda Creek without getting wet feet at 0.7 mile.

Turn right onto Canal Road at 0.9 mile, cross a creek on the roadway bridge, and turn left into the woods in 0.1 mile. Rise and descend over a low knob and cross a wooden bridge at 1.4 miles, coming onto the long boardwalk over Pochuck Swamp. The suspension bridge over Pochuck Creek is at 1.6 miles. Because of the unpredictable water levels, the bridge is constructed with a "floating" foundation that sits atop two large metal grids, crushed stone, and poured concrete—all underground and out of sight. According to one designer, it is built to hold 180 backpackers during a snowstorm with 18 inches of snow in a 70-mile-per-hour-wind. After the bridge, cross two more boardwalks—the first 1,000 feet long, the second 2,000 feet in length.

At 2.3 miles, cross County Road 517 and turn right to walk beside it for a few feet before leaving it to rise to the top of a low ridge at 2.9 miles. Descend and cross County Road 565 at 3.8 miles. Passing through swampy areas and overgrown fields, rise gradually to the summit of Pochuck Mountain (elevation 1,194 feet) at 5 miles. A side trail of about ten yards leads to a view across the western ridge of the mountain.

Cross a dirt road and some bog bridges in a swampy area at 5.2 miles. This may be the only source of water you will find on the mountain. Be sure to purify it before using. There is a pleasant view across the Wallkill Valley to High Point and the Kittatinny and Shawangunk Mountains from the end of a short rise at 5.7 miles. A short descent and another short ascent bring you to the top of Pochuck Mountain's western ridge before

you descend to the Pochuck Mountain Shelter side trail at 6.5 miles. Only 0.1 mile from the A.T, the shelter is the only place you are permitted to camp on this hike.

Continue to descend, soon passing through an open field with views to the west. At 7 miles, turn right onto Lake Wallkill Road and follow it for 40 yards before turning left to reenter the woods, soon using bog bridges across a wet area. Enter the Wallkill National Wildlife Refuge at 7.5 miles, and turn left onto a dirt road, which is also the refuge's Liberty Loop Trail. These lands were once a sod farm and you will pass by irrigation ditches and other evidence of earlier days. The A.T. will make two 90-degree turns before emerging onto Oil City Road at mile 9.

Turn left along the road, cross the Wallkill River on the highway bridge, and turn left onto a private road at 9.5 miles. Turn right to leave the road just 0.2 mile later and rise to the top of a small hill at 10.2 miles. Cross Oil City Road—different road, same name—at 10.3 miles, and New Jersey 284 at 10.8 miles. Turn right onto an old railroad grade at 11.1 miles. The railroad provided service on this line from around 1872 until 1958. Turn left and leave the railroad grade to follow a stone wall just 0.5 mile later. Soon, turn left into the woods and ascend slightly to Lott Road at 11.8 miles.

TRAILHEAD DIRECTIONS

A designated parking area for the northern trailhead is located on New Jersey 94, about 2.4 miles north of Vernon. For the southern trailhead, the A.T crosses Lott Road (Jersey Avenue), 0.4 mile south of New York 284 in Unionville. Although you may be able to find a space beside the road, you might want to consider leaving your car on a residential street in Unionville.

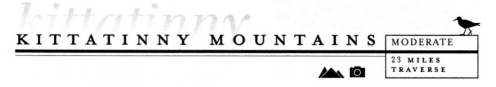

KITTATINNY MOUNTAINS

MODERATE

23 MILES
TRAVERSE

From the rolling farmlands, pastures, fields, and open woods of the Kittatinny Valley, this traverse takes you up along the ridge of the Kittatinny Mountains on a rocky footpath that passes through hickory and scrub oak forests. One of the highlights is High Point State Park, where the Appalachian Trail passes near the high point in the state of New Jersey. A short side trail (0.25 mile round-trip) leads from the A.T. to the summit (elevation 1,803 feet) with its stone monument.

THE HIKE

From the Appalachian Trail crossing on Lott Road (Jersey Avenue) south of Unionville, head south and ascend into the woods. There is a house visible to the right of the Trail. In 0.1 mile, you will enter an open field, head right across it for 0.1 mile, and enter the woods. You will climb gradually, while crossing a number of old quarry roads.

At mile 0.5, you will reach the crest of the hill, follow the left fork of the Trail, and descend. Just 0.2 mile later, you will reach Quarry Road; cross it, enter the woods on the other side, and pass an old quarry pit and a house on the right. At mile 0.9, reach Unionville Road (County 651). Cross the road diagonally to the left and enter the woods again.

In 0.1 mile, you will cross a stone wall as the Trail enters an open field. After ascending a hill, cross a farm road, continue on another farm road, turn left a short distance later, and pass through a field break. You will then walk through an old apple orchard and reach Goldsmith Lane at mile 1.4.

After crossing the lane, enter an overgrown successional field, and a short distance later, you will head right and cross a stone wall. In 0.1 mile, use more than 100 bog bridges to cross Vernie Swamp before reaching Goldsmith Road at mile 1.7. Cross the road, enter a field, and pass trees and a stone wall on your right that marks the New York–New Jersey border.

At the crest of Wolf Pit Hill (mile 1.9), enjoy a good view of High Point Monument straight ahead. A view of Pochuck Mountain is on the horizon behind you. From here, descend with pines to your right, and in 0.1 mile, pass a pond to your left, cross a concrete dam, and enter a field. Cross the field heading left, enter the woods, and climb up a gentle hill to the crest in 0.1 mile. Descend.

In 0.1 mile, you will reach Goodrich Road, cross it, take a short walk through the woods, and enter an overgrown field. You will soon cross three small streams, all of them on log bridges. Ascend and reach the crest of the ridge at mile 2.8, where you descend to pass through a muddy area at mile 2.9. Cross another stream, and reach an intersection of stone walls in another 0.1 mile. Turn right and enter a successional field scattered with cedars. Cross the field, bearing to the right.

In 0.1 mile, turn right, cross a brook, and then follow posts through an overgrown field. At mile 3.2, you will reach Gemmer Road; turn right, follow the road a short distance, turn left, and enter the woods. You will soon pass by a swampy area; shortly thereafter, cross a small brook, head right, and begin to climb, while passing through another swampy area.

Enter a field and follow the blazed posts. Cross a stone wall and reenter the woods. At mile 3.8, you will reach Ferguson Road. Turn right and follow the road a short distance before turning left and crossing a stile into another pasture. Follow the blazes across the pasture for 0.1 mile to a swampy area that you will cross on bog bridges. From there, cross over a stream on a bridge, turn left, and follow more blazed posts across a pasture while passing through another muddy area.

At an intersection of stone walls, turn right and cross a stile into a cultivated field. This land is currently being farmed under a lease agreement with its former owner, whose family has worked the land for several generations. Head around the edge of the field following the tree line to the left.

At the end of the field, in 0.1 mile, turn right but continue to follow the tree line to the left. You will soon cross a stone wall before turning left and skirting the field again. Follow the tree line to the left. The A.T. makes many twists and turns in this area, so be sure to follow the white blazes.

Around mile 4.8, follow the blazes across, and along, a number of old stone walls. You will reach Courtwright Road at mile 5. Cross the road and continue straight ahead into the woods. In 0.1 mile, cross a stream, and in another 0.1 mile, cross a grassy woods road and another stream before you enter an overgrown field.

Beyond the field, enter the woods (passing through a swampy area) and soon cross several stone walls. You will leave the woods 0.4 mile later and pass through fields, skirting to the right of some trees on the rise. At mile 5.8, you will reach County Road 519. After crossing the road (to the left), enter the woods and begin to climb on switchbacks.

In 0.2 mile, you will pass through a swampy area and enter an overgrown clearing. A short distance later, skirt fields through a swampy area, pass through breaks in several stone walls at the top of a ridge, turn left onto a dirt road, follow the road a short distance, and cross an intermittent stream at mile 6.8. At mile 7.1, a blue-blazed side trail continues straight ahead for 0.1 mile to High Point Shelter. Water is available from streams just before and just beyond the shelter.

Continue along the A.T. and reach another intersection in 0.5 mile. This blue-blazed side trail leads to High Point Monument, a 0.25-mile round-trip. Turn left to continue along the A.T. for 0.2 mile to reach a wooden observation platform, where there is an excellent panoramic view. Look east to view Kittatinny Valley with Pochuck Mountain in the foreground and Wawayanda Mountain on the horizon. Look southeast and you may be able to see the New York City skyline. Delaware Water Gap is to the southwest, and Lake Marcia and Highpoint Lodge with the Pocono Mountains of Pennsylvania are to the west. The Catskill Plateau is to the northwest, and High Point Monument is to the north.

The A.T. continues south along the ridge, passing through scrub, oak, and blueberry bushes. A short distance later, descend more steeply, then gradually again.

At mile 8.8, you will leave the woods and reach New Jersey 23. Cross the road, walk through a lawn by the driveway of High Point State Park Headquarters, and enter the woods at the south end of the parking lot. A short distance later, you will pass an unmarked trail that leads to a day-use parking area.

At mile 9, you will pass by the intersection with the red-on-white blazed Iris Trail, which comes in from the left. The yellow-blazed Mashipacong Trail, which has run concurrently with the A.T. since the south end of the parking lot, goes off to the right. Climb slightly for 0.1 mile, turn left onto an old woods road, and soon turn right, leaving the road and ascending to the ridge. When you reach the crest of the ridge, turn left and reach the junction of the Blue Dot Trail in 0.3 mile.

The A.T. reaches a viewpoint to the west over Sawmill Lake at 9.8 miles and then descends to the left into a mountain valley. Once you reach the valley floor, you will begin to ascend the next ridge to the east. Reach the top of the eastern ridge in 0.1 mile, and enjoy the view back over the valley with the distant Pocono Mountains visible to the left. The Trail crosses to the opposite side of the ridge and reaches the first in a series of viewpoints. Lake Rutherford can be seen below as the Trail continues along the ridge.

You will soon descend. At mile 10.7, turn right. At mile 11.2, enjoy another viewpoint from open rocks, and at mile 11.4 reach Dutch Shoe Rock with views to the northeast. A side trail leads left for 0.4 mile to the Rutherford Shelter. Water is available from a nearby spring.

The A.T. continues across large, open rocks before entering the woods and descending. After 0.5 mile, you will cross a stream and ascend. Turn right onto the red-on-white-blazed Iris Trail (a woods road) in 0.3 mile. To the left, the Iris Trail heads back to NJ 23. A short distance later, you will turn left off the Iris Trail and descend into a swampy area.

Hike 0.2 mile and ascend slightly before descending to another swampy area. Cross a stream at mile 12.6 and begin ascending again. In 0.1 mile, you will climb some rocks, turn right, and continue to climb more gradually. After crossing a cleared strip of land that contains a buried pipeline, you will reach a short side trail that leads to a view of farmland.

Sign the Trail register at mile 13.3, and continue past a private home on the left. Shortly thereafter, you will cross the Iris Trail again before beginning to descend. Cross rocks over a swampy area, and in another 0.2 mile, pass through another swampy area. Climb again.

At mile 14.1, you will reach the parking area on Deckertown Turnpike. Cross the road diagonally to the left and ascend to the Mashipacong Shelter, which is in a clearing. No water is available. The hand pump which used to supply water near the Deckertown Turnpike crossing has been removed.

The Trail reenters the woods on the far side to the right. In 0.7 mile, you will turn left onto Swenson Road (an old woods road), walk a short distance, turn right as the road curves left, and ascend. In 0.6 mile, you will skirt the top of the rise and begin to descend, passing through a mountain laurel thicket.

At the bottom of the descent, turn right and soon cross the outlet of a swamp to the left of the Trail. A short distance later, cross a stone wall and start to climb through a stand of white birches. You will reach the top of the hill at mile 16.2. Start to descend, soon crossing a stone wall, and reaching a rocky area 0.3 mile later.

From here, you will ascend to the top of a knoll, descend to Crigger Road, and ascend again. At mile 17.6, you will pass the parking area for Sunrise Mountain on your right. A short distance past the rest rooms, a path from the parking area joins the A.T. for the climb to the summit. It is barely 0.1 mile to the shelter atop the summit of Sunrise Mountain (elevation 1,653 feet); enjoy good views to the east and the west. Camping is not permitted at the shelter, which has a roof but no walls.

From the southeast corner of the shelter, descend a short distance and arrive on open ledges with beautiful views to the east. On the far side of the clearing, you will reenter the woods and descend, turning right along the rocks.

You will soon pass a viewpoint through the trees to the left as the Trail levels off and continues to descend gradually. After ascending over a knoll and then descending gradually, you will reach the intersection of the yellow-blazed Tinsley Trail at mile 18.7. The A.T. climbs a short distance before continuing along the western side of the ridge.

About 0.5 mile later, you will ascend and then descend gradually. Pass several ponds and swamps (when it is wet) to the left of the Trail. Shortly thereafter, you will pass through several more wet sections before reaching the blue-blazed Stony Brook Trail at mile 20.1. This trail leads 0.3 mile to the right to the Gren Anderson Shelter. Water is available from a spring a about 200 yards beyond the shelter.

Continuing along the A.T., cross Stony Brook in 0.1 mile. At mile 21.1, you will reach the green-blazed Tower Trail, which descends to the right. Sign the Trail register here. Following a brief climb 0.1 mile later, you will reach the Culver Fire Tower, which offers a wonderful 360-degree view for those willing to climb to the top. View Lake Owassa to the southwest, left of the Kittatinny Ridge, and view Kittatinny Lake to the right of the ridge. Much of this view is available to those who do not want to climb the tower.

The A.T. leaves the tower clearing from the southwest, turns right, and descends. Eventually, you will see Culver Lake through the trees to the left. Cross a small, grassy clearing 0.4 mile later, and reach a viewpoint, again somewhat obstructed by trees, over Culver Lake in another 0.5 mile.

Shortly thereafter, make a right turn and reach a viewpoint over Kittatinny Lake. The Trail turns right again and continues to descend, making a sharp left turn before reaching Sunrise Mountain Road at mile 22.7. Turn left and follow the road before reentering the woods. Soon come to the short trail to the parking area. Take that route and return to your car at mile 23.

Trailhead Directions

The A.T. crossing on Lott Road (Jersey Avenue) is 0.4 mile south of New York 284 in Unionville. Although you may be able to find a space beside the road, you might want to consider leaving your car on a residential street in Unionville.

Registration is required to park overnight at the southern trailhead, so follow US 206 northeast of Branchville, New Jersey to Culvers Gap. Continue another 0.5 mile to the Stokes State Forest office. After registering, return to Culvers Gap, turn left onto Upper North Shore Road and go another 0.3 mile to the parking area on Sunrise Mountain Road, just north of its intersection with Upper North Shore Road.

DELAWARE WATER GAP AND KITTATINNY MOUNTAINS

MODERATE

27 MILES
TRAVERSE

This hike begins in Delaware Water Gap near the Pennsylvania–New Jersey border, passes through the Worthington State Forest, and follows the Kittatinny Ridge to Culvers Gap. Among the highlights of this traverse are the beautiful glacier-cut Sunfish Pond and the wonderful views along the Kittatinny Ridge. A section of this hike passes through oak and hickory forests with scattered pitch pine, white pine, red cedar, hemlock, and rhododendrons. During midsummer, blueberries are plentiful along the Trail.

A dam was authorized to be built in the Delaware Water Gap area in 1962. Severe opposition halted the project, but not before the government established the Delaware Water Gap National Recreation Area, meant to provide recreational facilities for the never-established lake. The recreation area now provides a protected corridor for the Appalachian Trail.

Throughout much of this hike, camping is permitted only at shelters or designated campsites. Camping is permitted on the recreation area lands between mile 6.5 and mile 22.1. However, you must follow certain conditions: Camping is permitted only in areas that are 0.5 mile from road accesses or the boundaries of the national recreation area. You must camp not more than 100 feet from the Trail and at least 200 feet from other campsites. Camping is prohibited within 100 feet of any stream or water source. No camping is permitted from 0.5 mile south of Blue Mountain Lakes Road to 1 north of Crater Lake.

THE HIKE

From the Dunnfield Creek Natural Area, follow the A.T. north through the parking area, pass a pump with good water (it has been tested), and enter the woods. After turning left at mile 0.2, cross a wooden bridge over Dunnfield Creek, and shortly thereafter, turn right onto a woods road, following the left bank of Dunnfield Creek.

Take the left fork at mile 0.5 and continue along the woods road. The blue-blazed Blue Dot Trail leads right to Mount Tammany. Also at this intersection, the Dunnfield Creek Trail follows the route of the Blue Dot Trail for a distance before branching off to rise to Sunfish Pond. The A.T. continues to follow the woods roads as it gradually ascends. At mile 1.6, you will reach the junction with the yellow-blazed Beulahland Trail, which heads left to Fairview Parking Area on River Road. There is also the red-blazed Holly Spring Trail which goes right for 0.2 mile to intermittent Holly Spring.

The A.T. continues ahead with the Kittatinny Mountains visible to your right. At mile 2.6, pass by a grassy road which goes left to soon intersect the Douglas Trail. At mile 3.2, you will pass Backpacker Site (a designated camping site) at a trail junction. Turn right onto the woods road. To the left, the blue-blazed Douglas Trail leads 1.7 miles to a developed campground along the Delaware River in Worthington State Forest. The Trail is named for William O. Douglas, who campaigned against the proposed dam in the 1960s. He is also the only US Supreme Court Justice to have hiked the entire Appalachian Trail.

Hike 0.6 mile to Sunfish Pond. This glacial pond has been designated a Natural Area as well as a national landmark. Camping is not permitted here. The Trail skirts the pond and crosses its outlet and the Sunfish Drainage Trail at mile 4.1. Walking beside interesting rock formations, pass by the junction with the Turquoise Trail at mile 4.5 and, in another 0.1 mile, the yellow-blazed Garvey Trail, which leads left 0.1 mile to seasonal Garvey Springs. Descend to cross a brook, and reach a power line cut-through at mile 6.2, which provides views from both sides of the ridge. At the crest of the ridge, 0.1 mile later, you should be able to see the storage ponds for Yards Creek pump-storage hydroelectric development to the right and the Delaware River to the left. A view of Catfish Fire Tower lies ahead between the ridges.

Leave Worthington State Forest at mile 6.5 and enter the Delaware Water Gap National Recreation Area. After 0.2 mile, the overgrown Kaiser Road comes in from the right. In another 0.3 mile, the Kaiser Road Trail takes off to the left. Hike 0.4 mile to reach another viewpoint where you can get another eyeful of Yards Creek storage ponds. At mile 7.9, the Trail turns left, descends, and crosses a stream. (Red-blazed Coppermines Trail goes off to the left here.) Pick up water from the stream if you intend to camp along the first couple of miles atop the ridge. Reach Camp Road (formerly Mohican Road) at mile 8.9. From the far side of Camp Road, begin to ascend.

Climb 0.6 mile to the top of Kittatinny Ridge, and enjoy good views to the right. In another 0.6 mile or so, the Trail reaches the rim, follows the ledges a short distance, and reenters the woods. The ledges offer good views to the right. The Trail joins the rim again in another 0.1 mile. The orange-blazed Rattlesnake Swamp Trail heads left for 0.5 mile to Catfish Pond and the Mohican Outdoor Center. Hike another 1 mile to the Catfish Fire Tower, which offers a panoramic view from sixty feet above the ground. From the tower, you will begin your descent to Millbrook-Blairstown Road.

Follow the gravel road from the tower for 0.3 mile. Turn left off the road, and be sure to follow white blazes through a series of turns on and off gravel roads. Just after the orange-blazed Rattlesnake Swamp Trail intersects the gravel road you are following, you can take the gravel road to the left for 50 feet to Rattlesnake Spring, a reliable water source.

Continuing on the A.T., reach Millbrook-Blairstown Road at mile 12.3. Go left, following the paved road a short distance, and turn right onto a footpath. Cross a wooden bridge over a beaver pond outlet at mile 12.8. In 0.3 mile, reach a power line cut-through with views to the left of the Wallpack Valley and Pocono Plateau. Follow the cut-through to the right for 0.1 mile, turn left at the second power line tower, and enter the woods. A short side trail leads right to a view of Sand Pond of Camp No-Be-Bo-Sco, which belongs to the Bergen Council of the Boy Scouts of America.

The A.T follows the crest of the ridge through the woods. Pass by the side trail to the Boy Scout Camp in 0.8 mile. At mile 14.6, the A.T intersects a dirt road, which it follows for the next 1.6 miles. A clearing at mile 15.5 provides a view of Fairview Lake, while an unmarked road 0.4 mile later leads right 40 yards to a view of the lake and the highlands of New Jersey. Pass by a water pump (a good source of water as it is tested) and come to Blue Mountain Lakes Road at mile 16.2. Turn right to follow the road for 100 feet, turn left into the woods, and sign the Trail register 0.1 mile later. Cross the face of a smooth rock at mile 17.3, pass by a swamp at mile 17.5, and negotiate the face of a steep escarpment at mile 17.9. Intersect and turn right onto a gravel road at mile 18. Fifty feet later is a blue-blazed side trail to the right that goes 150 feet to a view of Crater Lake. Pass by orange-blazed Hemlock Trail in another 0.3 mile and the blue-blazed Buttermilk Falls Trail in an additional 0.8 mile. This latter pathway descend 1.6 miles and 1,000 feet in elevation to the falls—the highest in New Jersey.

Continuing on the A.T., leave the gravel road at mile 19.4, passing by an unmarked trail to the left (leads a distance to a western-looking view). After a descent, cross a stream at mile 20.6, where a blue-blazed side trail leads right to a water source. Rise to the top of Rattlesnake Mountain (elevation 1,492 feet) in another 0.4 mile, where you can look westward to the Wallpack Valley and the Pocono Plateau.

Cross a stream 0.3 mile later, turning right onto a dirt road in another 0.5 mile. Just after this is a unmarked trail to a view to the west. At mile 22.1, turn right off the dirt road and enter Stokes State Forest. In 0.4 mile, come into a clearing with a view of the Wallpack Valley and Pocono Plateau in Pennsylvania. Cross dirt Brink Road at mile 23.2. A blue-blazed side trail to the left goes 0.2 mile to Brink Road Shelter. Water is available about 100 yards beyond the shelter.

Continuing on the A.T., sign the Trail register at mile 23.6. An unmarked side trail at mile 24.7 goes to an overlook of Lake Owassa. Blue/gray–blazed Jacob's Ladder Trail descends to the left 0.2 mile later.

Another 0.7 mile brings you to a large cleared area with Culver Lake visible to the north and the Culver Fire Tower visible further north on the ridgeline you have been following. Make a right-angle turn in an additional 0.4 mile, where you have a view onto US 206 passing through Culvers Gap.

Cross over a gravel road (which is the route of the gold/brown-blazed Acropolis Trail) and under a power line at mile 26.3. Descend into Culvers Gap at the intersection of US 206 and Upper North Shore Road at mile 26.8. Cross the intersection, enter the woods and go another 0.2 mile to the short route to the parking area.

TRAILHEAD DIRECTIONS

The parking lot of the Dunnfield Creek Natural Area is located in Delaware Water Gap National Recreation Area. The recreation area is the first exit after crossing the I-80 toll bridge from Pennsylvania into New Jersey in the Delaware Water Gap. For those driving westward on I-80, the exit is the rest area just before the toll bridge. You will see the white-blazed A.T. as you pass by the information center. Follow the blazes as you drive to the parking lot at the trailhead, which is 0.5 mile beyond the information center.

Registration is required to park overnight at the northern trailhead, so follow US 206 northeast of Branchville, New Jersey to Culvers Gap. Continue another 0.5 mile to the Stokes State Forest office. After registering, return to Culvers Gap, turn left onto Upper North Shore Road and go another 0.3 mile to the parking area on Sunrise Mountain Road, just north of its intersection with Upper North Shore Road.

With close to 230 miles to traverse, the Appalachian Trail in Pennsylvania is both one of the easiest and hardest to hike. The Trail is often characterized by a tough climb up a ridge followed by a level, but rocky walk.

The A.T. begins in Pennsylvania at the Delaware Water Gap in the Kittatinny Mountains, where it climbs more than 1,000 feet to the summit of Mount Minsi.

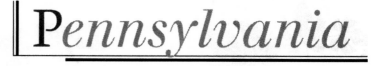

Pennsylvania

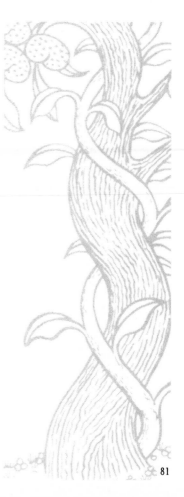

This rough and rocky trail then traverses the ridge from gap to gap (Totts, Fox, Wind, Smith, Little, and finally the rocky face of Lehigh Gap).

For the next 30 miles (after you climb out of Lehigh Gap), the Trail once again follows the ridge, passing Bake Oven Knob, The Cliffs, and Blue Mountain Summit before reaching the area of Hawk Mountain Sanctuary near Eckville. From here, the Trail climbs once again to the ridge, passing The Pinnacle, an outstanding viewpoint over the Pennsylvania countryside.

From The Pinnacle, the A.T. drops down to Windsor Furnace, the site of an old iron stove plant; glassy slag can still be seen along the Trail. The A.T. continues to Port Clinton

WHERE IT REGAINS THE RIDGE AND FOL-
LOWS IT FOR MORE THAN 30 MILES. FROM
SWATARA GAP, THE TRAIL LEAVES BLUE
MOUNTAIN, CROSSES ST. ANTHONY'S
WILDERNESS, AND PASSES THE SITES OF
RAUSCH GAP AND YELLOW GAP VILLAGES.
AFTER ASCENDING SECOND MOUNTAIN,
SHARP MOUNTAIN, AND STONY MOUN-
TAIN, THE TRAIL CLIMBS TO THE RIDGE OF
PETERS MOUNTAIN AND FOLLOWS IT FOR
15 MILES BEFORE DESCENDING TO THE
SUSQUEHANNA RIVER AT DUNCANNON,
PENNSYLVANIA.

THE A.T. HEADS SOUTHWEST AT THE
SUSQUEHANNA, CROSSING COVE AND BLUE
MOUNTAINS AND FALLING TO THE CUM-
BERLAND VALLEY. THIS AREA OF THE TRAIL
WAS ONCE FAMOUS FOR ITS LONG ROAD
WALK, BUT THE TRAIL HAS NOW BEEN
REROUTED OFF ROADS THROUGH WOODS
AND ROLLING FARMLAND. AT THE END OF
THE VALLEY, THE TRAIL CLIMBS SOUTH
MOUNTAIN, WHICH IT FOLLOWS ALL THE
WAY THROUGH MARYLAND.

THE SOUTHERN SECTION OF TRAIL IN
PENNSYLVANIA PASSES THROUGH THE VIL-
LAGE OF BOILING SPRINGS WITH ITS BEAU-
TIFUL CHILDREN'S LAKE, PINE GROVE
FURNACE STATE PARK WITH ITS MODEL

FURNACE AND IRONMASTER'S MANSION,
AND CALEDONIA STATE PARK WITH THE
THADDEUS STEVENS MUSEUM BEFORE IT
REACHES THE PENNSYLVANIA–MARYLAND
STATE LINE.

WITH CLOSE TO 230 MILES TO TRAVERSE,
THE APPALACHIAN TRAIL IN PENNSYLVA-
NIA VARIES IN DIFFICULTY AND IS OFTEN
CHARACTERIZED BY A TOUGH CLIMB UP A
RIDGE FOLLOWED BY A LEVEL, BUT ROCKY
WALK.

THE TRAIL BEGINS IN PENNSYLVANIA AT
THE DELAWARE WATER GAP WHERE IT
CLIMBS MORE THAN 1,000 FEET TO THE
SUMMIT OF MOUNT MINSI. THE TRAIL
PASSES BAKE OVEN KNOB, THE CLIFFS, AND
BLUE MOUNTAIN SUMMIT AND REACHES
THE AREA OF HAWK MOUNTAIN SANCTUARY.

FROM HERE, THE TRAIL CLIMBS AGAIN TO
THE RIDGE, AND PASSES THE PINNACLE
NEAR ECKVILLE, DROPS DOWN TO WIND-
SOR FURNACE, AND CONTINUES TO PORT
CLINTON. FROM SWATARA GAP, THE
TRAIL LEAVES BLUE MOUNTAIN, CROSSES
ST. ANTHONY'S WILDERNESS, AND PASSES
THE SITES OF RAUSCH GAP AND YELLOW
GAP VILLAGES. AFTER ASCENDING SEC-
OND, SHARP, AND STONY MOUNTAINS,

THE A.T. CLIMBS TO THE RIDGE OF PETERS MOUNTAIN BEFORE DESCENDING TO THE SUSQUEHANNA RIVER AT DUNCANNON. THE TRAIL HEADS SOUTHWEST AT THE SUSQUEHANNA, CROSSING COVE AND BLUE MOUNTAINS AND FALLING TO THE CUMBERLAND VALLEY. AT THE END OF THE VALLEY, THE TRAIL CLIMBS SOUTH MOUNTAIN. THE SOUTHERN SECTION OF TRAIL IN PENNSYLVANIA PASSES THROUGH THE VILLAGE OF BOILING SPRINGS AND CALEDONIA STATE PARK BEFORE IT REACHES THE PENNSYLVANIA–MARYLAND STATE LINE.

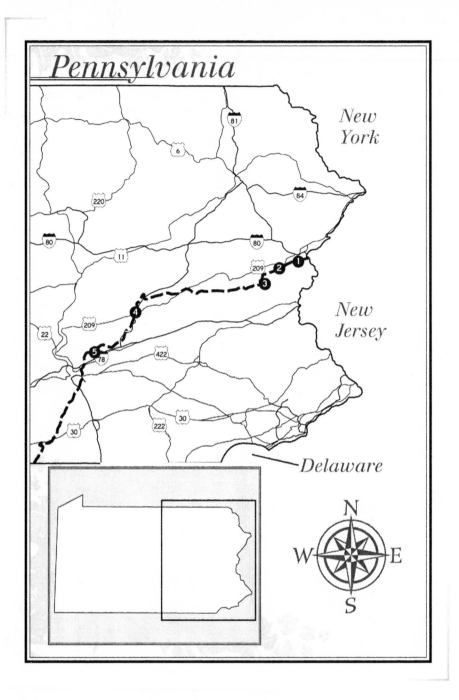

Pennsylvania

New York

New Jersey

Delaware

N
W E
S

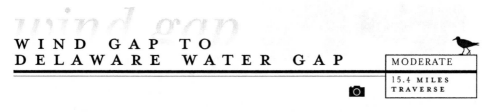

WIND GAP TO
DELAWARE WATER GAP

MODERATE

15.4 MILES
TRAVERSE

This hike features a number of good views as it rambles over the Kittatinny Ridge in Pennsylvania. From Wind Gap, it is a rocky but beautiful hike to Delaware Water Gap. The club members that maintain this section joke that they sharpen the rocks each spring in anticipation of the year's hikers. Make sure you're wearing sturdy boots with lots of ankle support! Also, if you're hiking during late summer, remember that water is scarce in this section, so bring plenty with you.

Highlights of this hike include Wolf Rocks, Lookout Rock, Council Rock, and Lake Lenape. Keep an eye out at Wolf Rocks for the white blazes that mark the A.T. because the mountain is nearly a mile wide at this point, and it is easy to get lost amid the massive, tumbled boulders that cover the area. These huge boulders, covered with rock tripe and lichens, offer great views of the surrounding countryside. At Council Rock, look for the profile of Chief Tammany on the opposite mountain across the Delaware River.

THE HIKE

An official A.T. signboard marks the beginning of the hike. From the road at Wind Gap, climb steeply up through the woods. At mile 2.1, cross the Blue Mountain Water Company Road, enjoy the good views, and continue to the top of the ridge.

Follow the ridge, where at mile 6.5, reach Wolf Rocks, with a view ahead to Fox Gap along Blue Mountain to Delaware Water Gap; on clear days you can see the Kittatinny Ridge in New Jersey. The Trail turns right onto Wolf Rocks before turning left and dropping off the north side of the rocks.

Continue along the ridge for another 0.3 mile, and reach an old road on the left that comes up the mountain from Cherry Valley. Take a right on this road and pass under a power line. At mile 7.7, the Trail turns left off the road and reenters the woods. Pass under a telephone cable and enjoy a good view of Stroudsburg to the north at mile 8.4.

Reach Fox Gap at Pennsylvania 191 in 0.2 mile. Cross the road, hike 0.1 mile to cross a green-blazed pathway. Another 0.3 mile brings you to the junction with the orange-blazed "Great Walk," which descends 0.8 mile to a reproduction of an early Celtic Christian Church. A blue-blazed trail at mile 9.3 goes a short distance to Kirkridge Shelter, with a nice south-facing view. Water is available beyond the shelter a short distance along a blue-blazed trail. This faucet is the property of the Kirkridge Retreat; hikers are allowed to use the spigot. Turn the water off when finished.

Continue on the A.T. for 0.1 mile to cross a gravel road. Lunch Rocks, with a view into New Jersey, is passed in another 0.6 mile. Continue on the ridge, crossing under two sets of power lines at mile 10.9. Descend a rocky trail for 0.1 mile to Totts Gap.

At the gap, the Trail heads right into the woods and passes several communications towers. At mile 11.3, the Trail turns left before turning right onto a gravel road. The A.T. follows the road for 1.7 miles to a side trail to the right that leads 100 feet to a view of the Delaware River. Continue on the A.T. for 0.1 mile to the summit of Mount Minsi (elevation 1,480 feet). From the summit, descend on a series of switchbacks, where you'll have wonderful views of Delaware Water Gap.

Enjoy a view of the Pocono Plateau from the top of the rocks at mile 14. Descend via switchbacks and pass a short side trail to Lookout Rock at mile 14.1. Cross Eureka Creek in a rhododendron grove. At mile 14.9, you will reach Council Rock. Across the river, view the exposed rock face of Mount Tammany, which forms the shape of Chief Tammany's profile. Pass by a side trail in a hemlock grove, and reach a gravel road 0.2 mile later. From here, turn right downhill, arriving at pretty Lake Lenape at mile 15.4. There is a parking lot here where you can either leave a vehicle or be picked up.

TRAILHEAD DIRECTIONS

There is an entrance ramp onto Pennsylvania 33 in Wind Gap, but no exit. To get to the trailhead, take PA 33 to the town of Wind Gap. Take the main road north out of Wind Gap, and look for a well-marked parking area about a mile beyond the center of town.

The end of the hike is the parking lot at Lake Lenape, which can be reached from Pennsylvania 611 in Delaware Water Gap. Take Mountain Road, and the first fork to your left passes the parking area at Lake Lenape.

BLUE MOUNTAIN

MODERATE

13.3 MILES
TRAVERSE

This is one of the more scenic hikes in Pennsylvania. The Trail traverses Blue Mountain from Pennsylvania 309 at Blue Mountain Summit to Lehigh Gap. There are a number of highlights, including views from The Cliffs and Bear Rocks, and bird-watching from Bake Oven Knob. In the fall, the vantage point from Bake Oven Knob is great for those interested in following raptor migrations. Near the end of this hike, the North Trail (at its northernmost junction with the A.T.) leads a short distance to Devil's Pulpit and views overlooking the Lehigh River.

THE HIKE

Follow the blue-blazed trail from the parking lot, and hike north along the A.T., joining a woods road in 0.2 mile. Rise to the ridgeline and walk under a power line cut-through at mile 1.8. On the other side of the cut-through, the road becomes a rocky footpath. A blue-blazed side trail to the left descends 0.2 mile to the base of the valley and then beyond to New Tripoli Campsite. Water is available from a spring at the campsite.

Continue along the A.T., turn left at mile 2.9, and follow the knife-edged ridge called The Cliffs, where there is a view of Bear Rocks. Reach the blue-blazed side trail to Bear Rocks in another 0.6 mile. The side trail climbs a short distance to Bear Rocks, offering a 360-degree view of the Pennsylvania countryside.

Hike 1 mile and take the right fork at a grassy road. Reach Bake Oven Knob Road at mile 4.9. This cross-mountain gravel road is passable by vehicles, and there are often a number of cars parked in the game commission parking lot-people out day hiking, bird-watching, or partying.

In another 0.4 mile, you will pass over the summit of Bake Oven Knob (elevation 1,560 feet). The summit still bears the remains of an old airplane beacon. Look right for an outstanding, 180-degree view to the south, and left for views to the north. In the fall, this vantage point is great for bird-watchers interested in following hawk and other raptor migrations.

Continue along the A.T. and reach a rock slide on the mountain's north side. Cross with care. At mile 5.9, you will reach the Bake Oven Knob Shelter to the right of the Trail. A blue-blazed side trail at the shelter leads downhill to a spring (often dry) on the right, and a couple hundred yards farther to a more reliable spring, also on the right. The side trail continues another 0.75 mile to Bake Oven Knob Road. This road leads (to the left) another 1.1 miles to a paved road in the valley.

From the Bake Oven Knob Shelter, hike 0.8 mile to a good wintertime view to the north. The Trail follows a rock outcropping here and crosses a rocky crest on the north side of the mountain in 0.2 mile. At mile 8, pass under a transmission line and head right on Ashfield Road. A short distance later, you will pass a woods road with a gate; turn left into the woods. The Trail turns right 0.3 mile later and follows a boundary line for the Pennsylvania Game Lands (the boundary is also marked with white blazes, but unlike A.T. blazes, they are irregular in shape, size, and location).

At mile 9.3, the Trail turns left, away from the game lands boundary, and crosses an abandoned telephone line cut-through. Follow a rough trail to the top of some rocks, and enjoy superb views of the area. One mile after turning away from the game lands, you will pass over the Northeast Extension of the Pennsylvania Turnpike, which passes through a tunnel, unseen far below your feet.

You will meet the southern junction of the North Trail at mile 11.1. The North Trail is the more scenic route of the two trails, but it is vulnerable to winter storms. (From this southern junction, the North Trail leads 2 miles to a side trail that takes you downhill for 0.4 mile to the Devil's Pulpit, a rock outcropping with great views of Lehigh Gap. Continuing on the North Trail, it is 0.4 mile from the side trail to the A.T.)

From the southern junction of the North Trail, continue along the A.T., and hike along the southeast side of the mountain, reaching the northern junction of the North Trail in 1.5 miles. (From here, it is 0.4 mile on the North Trail to the side trail that leads another 0.4 mile downhill to Devil's Pulpit).

Hike 0.1 mile past the junction with the North Trail, and reach the George W. Outerbridge Shelter, and one of the best springs in Pennsylvania, especially appreciated on this water-scarce ridge. The piped spring nearly always gushes forth cold water and is on the A.T. a short distance past the shelter. The Trail passes by the shelter and descends past the spring. Just 0.4 mile after leaving the shelter, pass under power lines, where there are views of Lehigh Gap.

Hike 0.2 mile and reach the west end of the highway bridge (Pennsylvania 873) over the Lehigh River, the end of the traverse.

TRAILHEAD DIRECTIONS

The Trail crossing at Blue Mountain Summit can be reached by traveling south from Snyders on Pennsylvania 309. Parking is available in a game commission parking lot just north of the A.T. The hike ends at Pennsylvania 873/248 on the south side of the bridge, 2 miles south of Palmerton. Limited parking is available.

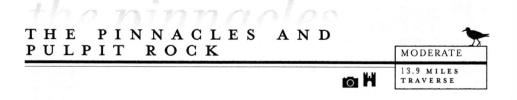

THE PINNACLES AND PULPIT ROCK

MODERATE

13.9 MILES
TRAVERSE

This traverse follows the ridge of Blue Mountain from Hawk Mountain Road near Eckville to The Pinnacles, Pulpit Rock, and down to Windsor Furnace and the town of Port Clinton. Views of the Pennsylvania farmland are spectacular from The Pinnacles, and Pulpit Rock offers splendid views of Blue Rocks, a stretch of jumbled boulders a mile long. Deposited during the glacial period, this 40,000-year-old sandstone rock gets its name from the quartzite and other minerals that give the stones a bluish tinge in early morning light and on moonlit evenings.

At Windsor Furnace, the site of an early pig-ironworks, glassy slag can still be seen in the pathway. Look for the remains of the old engine foundation in the undergrowth. Iron stoves were once manufactured at this furnace, and, interestingly, an iron replica of the Last Supper. The furnace was fueled by charcoal, and many charcoal hearths, 30 to 50 feet in diameter, can be seen on this hike, including a hearth at Pocahontas Spring.

THE HIKE

From the parking area off Hawk Mountain Road, a blue-blazed side trail leads 0.4 mile to the A.T. Turn left, head south on the A.T., and you will reach Panther Spring in 0.9 mile as you ascend the ridge. The spring to your right is a reliable water source.

One mile past the spring, at the junction of a woods road, the A.T. stays to the left. At mile 2.8, you will pass Gold Spring. This, too, is a reliable water source and is a short distance off the Trail to your right. Because it is part of the Hamburg Borough Watershed, camping and fires (unless otherwise noted) are not allowed in this area.

Continue along the A.T. and keep to your left where the woods road bears right,

0.3 mile past the spring. In another 0.75 mile, go left as the woods road bears right. In another 0.25 mile, when you reach a clearing, keep to the left again.

At mile 4.6, you will pass a charcoal hearth. In another 0.2 mile, you will reach the side trail leading to The Pinnacles. This short trail heads left to one of the most outstanding views in Pennsylvania. The Pinnacles (elevation 1,635 feet) looks out over the quilt-like landscape of Pennsylvania farmland. There are two caves to explore below The Pinnacles as well as many sheer cliffs. Keep an eye out for copperheads. No camping or fires are allowed here.

Continue along the A.T. to yellow-blazed side trail that leads to Blue Rocks at mile 5.2. This side trail heads left, often steeply, downhill for 1.3 miles to Blue Rocks, and another 0.2 to Blue Rocks Campground, which is privately owned. Continue along at the A.T. for another 1.1 miles, and cross a rock field, passing through a cleft in a rock formation in another 0.1 mile. Pass a rock field to our right in another 0.1 mile where there are good views to the north.

Enjoy excellent views to your left from a rock outcropping in 0.3 mile, and pass a tower to your right in another 0.1 mile. Reach Pulpit Rock (elevation 1,582 feet) 0.1 mile later. From Pulpit Rock, look left for wonderful views of The Pinnacles with Blue Rocks in the foreground.

Continue along the A.T. and pass the Astronomical Park of Lehigh Valley Amateur Astronomical Society. Hike another 0.1 mile along the A.T. to where the Trail heads left and descends the mountain along an old woods road. The blue-blazed trail to the left at mile 7.5 leads to privately-owned Blue Rocks Campground.

At mile 8.6, you will reach the side trail to Windsor Furnace Shelter. The blue-blazed trail heads right a short distance to the shelter and camping area. Questionable water is available from a creek.

After 0.1 mile, the Trail, now on a road, crosses Furnace Creek. Swimming and bathing are not allowed in the creek. Reach Windsor Furnace 0.1 mile past the creek. The Borough of Hamburg has provided a camping area about 500 yards south on a blue-blazed trail. The sites are just beyond the reservoir buildings on a dirt road to the left. A stream at the campsites provides water.

From the furnace, the A.T. continues to the left on an old woods road. At mile 9.4, take the right fork away from the woods road. In another 0.8 mile, you will pass an intermittent spring (almost always dry in the summer), and 1.2 miles later, you will reach Pocahontas Spring, which usually runs year-round. Camping is allowed in the vicinity of the spring. A blue-blazed trail here heads left 1 mile to the YMCA Blue Mountain Camp.

From Pocahontas Spring, hike 0.2 mile to the ridge and head left. In 0.7 mile, you will cross a telephone line cut-through, and in another 0.2 mile, a boundary line designating game lands. Reach the top of the ridge, where there are views of the Schuylkill River Valley and Dam.

At 13.3 miles, you will begin to descend the ridge on switchbacks. Reach the road crossing and parking area at mile 13.9, the end of the traverse.

TRAILHEAD DIRECTIONS

Just 0.5 mile south of Eckville, the unimproved Pine Swamp Road heads south to a Game Commission parking area on the right. A blue-blazed trail leads to the A.T. To reach Eckville, on Hawk Mountain Road, travel on Pennsylvania 895 from Drehersville or on Pennsylvania 143 near Kempton and Albany.

From Hamburg on Pennsylvania 61, parking is available a half-mile south of Port Clinton on a paved side road to your right.

HAWK ROCK AND THE CUMBERLAND VALLEY

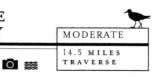

MODERATE

14.5 MILES
TRAVERSE

A steep, but short climb to Hawk Rock—sadly often covered by graffiti—provides a grandstand view of the Susquehanna River landscape. Directly below is Sherman Creek coursing eastward, while the Little Juniata River comes flowing in from the north. To the northeast are the homes and businesses of Duncannon, bordered by the waters of the Susquehanna River, which has widened considerably from its humble beginnings near Cooperstown, New York. A little more than 440 miles long, the Susquehanna is one of the longest rivers passed by the route of the A.T. from Georgia to Maine.

Beyond the jutting outcrop, the A.T. runs along the crest of Cove Mountain, where a pipeline right-of-way opens up another vista of the countryside before descending into a gap and rising over Little Mountain. The final short climb is over Blue Mountain. This is the same ridgeline the A.T. has coursed along since the Trail entered Pennsylvania at the Delaware Water Gap.

The last part of the hike is in the Cumberland Valley, a part of the Great Valley that stretches from Alabama to Canada. The A.T. crosses this natural travel conduit again in central and southern Virginia. Prior to land acquisitions by the National Park Service in the 1980s, the Trail was mostly a roadwalk through the Cumberland Valley. You will only be trekking in the valley for 2 miles, but the A.T.'s 14-mile traverse of it is now a pleasant walk along a low ridge, into open fields, and through the small village of Boiling Springs.

The Hike

Follow the A.T south from Susquehanna Avenue, rising quickly onto the northern slope of Cove Mountain. Cross over a prominent point and join an old woods road at 0.5 mile. The roadbed comes to an end where you cross a rockslide at 1 mile and the A.T. continues along a pathway. Reach Hawk Rock and its nice vista at 1.3 miles.

Having gained almost all of the elevation it is going to on Cove Mountain, the A.T. continues its traverse of the ridgeline with just very minor ups and downs. The blue-blazed trail to the left at 3.2 miles drops 0.1 mile to Cove Mountain Shelter and another 0.1 mile to a spring. The shelter was built in 2000 with timber and boards salvaged from a barn more than 100 years old.

Continue on the A.T., and pass by a side trail at 4.1 miles that descends right to a service road for the local water company. A pipeline right-of-way at 5.7 miles lets you gaze onto the Susquehanna River to one side of the mountain, while rural lands recede into the distance from the other side. An unmarked trail descends right to a Pennsylvania Game Commission parking lot.

Soon after beginning the gradual descent of the mountain, you will cross a stream at 6.8 miles. You should consider picking up (and treating) water here if you plan to spend the night at Darlington Shelter; its water source is often dry. Follow the white blazes of the A.T. to negotiate several turns and cross over Pennsylvania 850 at 8.2 miles. Gradually rise through a farm field, crossing Miller Gap Road in 0.4 mile. Turn left into a wooded ravine in another 0.1 mile, soon rising to cross over the high point on Little Mountain and descending to turn right onto a woods road at 9.6 miles.

At 10.2 miles, follow the A.T. as it turns left and ascends to the side trail for Darlington Shelter at 10.5 miles. The shelter is 0.1 mile from the A.T., while its spring is more than 0.2 mile beyond the shelter.

Continue on the A.T. and pass a major intersection at 10.6 miles. Orange-blazed Darlington Trail follows the jeep road to the left. Blue-blazed Tuscarora Trail, which runs close to 250 miles to Shenandoah National Park in Virginia, goes off to the right.

A rock outcrop at 10.9 miles provides a view of your final destination, the Cumberland Valley. Turn right onto a woods road at 11.2 miles, only to leave it by turning left in another 0.1 mile. Cross an old dirt road at 11.5 miles. There is a piped spring 50 feet to the right, and because cars move at high rates of speed, make a quick dash across Pennsylvania 944 (Wertzville Road) at 12.5 miles.

Stroll through the woodlands of the northern part of the Cumberland Valley and, at 13.4 miles, follow paved Sherwood Road for 0.1 mile before reentering the woods to walk beside Conodoguinet Creek. This can be an easy and pleasant ramble along the stream, but be mindful of the copious amounts of poison ivy. Reach the Scott Farm and the end of the hike at 14.5 miles.

TRAILHEAD DIRECTIONS

For the northern trailhead, follow Market Street south through Duncannon, pass under US 11/15, and at the intersection with Pennsylvania 274, turn left onto Susquehanna Avenue. Look for a parking space soon after crossing the Sherman Creek Bridge, or park at the end of the roadway.

For the southern trailhead, take I-81 Exit 17, and go west on US 11, but almost immediately turn right onto Country Club Road. Turn left onto Bernhisel Road, and immediately after crossing Conodoguinet Creek pull into the parking lot for the Appalachian Trail Conservancy's Scott Farm Trail Work Center. Let someone know you will be leaving your car overnight.

SOUTH MOUNTAIN

EASY

20.3 MILES TRAVERSE

The highlights of this hike include the preserved ruins of the iron furnace and the former Ironmaster's mansion at Pine Grove Furnace State Park and the iron furnace and museum at Caledonia State Park. From Pine Grove Furnace State Park, the A.T. ascends the ridge of South Mountain and follows the ridge until the descent to Caledonia State Park.

Pine Grove Furnace was owned by the Eges family that owned the furnace at Boiling Springs (also on the A.T.). The furnace produced firearms for the revolution in the late eighteenth century. The furnace was later purchased by the Watts family, and by the mid-1800s included the furnace, a forge, coal house, brick mansion, smith and carpenter shops, 30 log dwellings, and grist- and saw-mills. The 35,000 acres surrounding the furnace were exploited to get charcoal to fuel the furnace. All structures except the mansion and furnace were destroyed in a 1915 fire. A small museum features the natural and industrial history of the area.

George and Martha Washington are said to have stayed at the Ironmaster's home during the wedding of the Ironmaster's daughter. The Ironmaster's daughter, upon the birth of twins (male and female), gave the president and first lady the honor of naming her children. They graced the pair with the names of George and Martha. The ironworks finally closed in 1893, having operated since 1762.

The railroad that once serviced the furnaces in the area is now a roadbed, part of which is used by the Appalachian Trail. While sharing the old railbed, the A.T. passes Fuller Lake. The lake, which is about 90 feet deep, was the ore hole for the furnace. When the pumps broke down at the turn of the century, the mine was flooded and abandoned; the lake remains.

The A.T. also passes the mansion, which is now an American Youth Hostel. Also along the Trail in this area, you'll find traces of the old charcoal hearths, 30 to 50 feet in diameter, and the bluish-green glassy slag from the furnace.

Caledonia State Park also features one of the ten iron furnaces in the South Mountain area. Caledonia's furnace was built in 1837, and was owned by abolitionist Thaddeus Stevens at the time of the Civil War. His ironworks was destroyed by the Confederate Army en route to the Battle of Gettysburg. Only the furnace and the old blacksmith shop remain. The blacksmith shop, which

sat along a former A.T. route, is now a museum. The old A.T. route is now a blue-blazed trail that leads to the museum as well as a swimming pool and concession area.

You will also pass the site of the former Camp Michaux. Take the time to locate the ruins of a large stone barn. The Keystone Trails Association used to hold its fall meeting at this former church camp. The site was also once a prisoner-of-war camp for captured German submarine crews. Before the war, it served as a CCC camp.

THE HIKE

The Trail crossing at Pine Grove Furnace State Park can be picked up in the park near the store and mansion, or from Pennsylvania 233 that is about 500 yards west of the park. The Trail heads south on a gravel road. The gravel road ends in 0.1 mile, and the A.T. enters an old woods road.

At mile 0.7, you will leave the woods road and pass several charcoal flats. In another 0.6 mile, you will pass the intersection of the blue-blazed Sunset Rocks Trail to your left. The Trail heads 2.4 miles to the Toms Run Shelters.

Hike 0.1 mile, cross Toms Run on a foot-bridge, then turn left onto the Old Shippensburg Road. At mile 1.6, you will reach a side trail that leads a short distance to Half Way Spring. From here, hike 0.4 mile to a clearing, which is the site of the former Camp Michaux. Locate the ruins of a large stone barn.

At the former camp site, the Trail turns right onto Michaux Road. Hike 0.2 mile and turn left onto a gated woods road. At mile 3.4, you will reach Toms Run Shelters, twin shelters rebuilt in 1992. Water is available from a spring behind the old chimney. You will cross Toms Run again and reach the southern junction of the Sunset Rocks Trail to your left. From here, the A.T. climbs steeply.

At mile 4.6, cross Woodrow Road, after an additional 0.6 mile you will turn right and parallel Ridge Road, which is a short distance to your right.

In 1.4 miles, reach the junction with a blue-blazed side trail that leads to the Anna Michener Memorial Cabin—belonging to the Potomac Appalachian Trail Club—the Dead Woman Hollow Trail, and the Blueberry Trail. At mile 7.3, after arriving at the crest of the hill, the A.T. crosses the old roadbed of Dead Woman Hollow Road, which is now a winter snowmobile trail.

Just 1 mile later, you will cross the Arendtsville-Shippensburg Road.

Hike 1.4 miles to Birch Run and the Birch Run Shelters at mile 9.7. Cross Birch Run. Water is available from a spring to the right of the shelters. Continue along the A.T., cross the old Fegley Hollow Road in 0.6 mile. Hike another 0.7 mile to Michaux Forest's Rocky Knob Trail on the left. Ridge Road is a short distance to the right; you will cross it in 0.7 mile and begin to descend steeply.

You will cross Milesburn Road at mile 12.1. The PATC's Milesburn Cabin is just ahead. A blue-blazed trail leads right downstream and across Milesburn Road to a spring. The Trail begins to climb steeply.

In another 0.4 mile, you will reach the intersection of Canada Hollow Road, Means Hollow Road, and Ridge Road. After crossing the roads, hike 0.4 mile to pass Dughill Trail; 0.1 mile later, you will cross Middle Ridge Road. Once again, the Trail parallels Ridge Road.

At mile 15.6, you will reach the intersection of Ridge Road and Stillhouse Road in an area called Sandy Sod. The Trail follows Ridge Road for 0.1 mile, turns left into the woods, and descends through Quarry Gap. In another 0.7 mile, you will reach the junction of the Hosack Run Trail on your left. The Hosack Run Trail connects with the Locust Gap Trail in 1.1 miles.

The A.T. turns left after 0.5 mile where an intermittent stream comes in from the right and follows the stream downhill, arriving at Quarry Gap Shelters in 0.2 mile. The two shelters at Quarry Gap were rebuilt in 1993. Water is available from a small spring that feeds the creek.

Continue on the A.T. and pass another spring in 0.4 mile. The spring is near the site of the former Antlers Camp. There is a gate here to control access to the Quarry Gap Shelters.

After 0.3 mile, turn right onto Greenwood Furnace Road; the blue-blazed Locust Gap Trail enters from the left on Greenwood Road. This trail leads left 1.8 miles to Milesburn Road. Continue along the A.T./Locust Gap Trail and take the left fork at a former rifle range, then climb steeply up Chinquapin Hill. The Locust Gap Trail now continues ahead 3 miles to Houser Road and Fayetteville near US 30. Follow the A.T. left and pass the blue-blazed Caledonia Park Three Valley Trail.

You will pass two parking lots. A rest room that is open year-round adjoins the second lot. The road goes to the park office. Hike another 1.4 miles and cross Conococheague Creek on Caledonia Park bridge. Follow the A.T. right, where the former A.T., now blue-blazed, goes left and passes the park swimming pool and museum. The new A.T. crosses a bridge over a former canal in 0.2 mile and reaches US 30, only 0.1 mile later. Walk 0.6 mile east (left) to the parking area off PA 233 at Caledonia State Park, which is the end of the traverse.

Trailhead Directions

Parking is available at Pine Grove Furnace State Park off PA 233. Caledonia State Park is also located on PA 233.

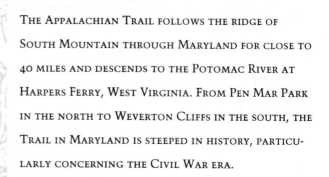

THE APPALACHIAN TRAIL FOLLOWS THE RIDGE OF SOUTH MOUNTAIN THROUGH MARYLAND FOR CLOSE TO 40 MILES AND DESCENDS TO THE POTOMAC RIVER AT HARPERS FERRY, WEST VIRGINIA. FROM PEN MAR PARK IN THE NORTH TO WEVERTON CLIFFS IN THE SOUTH, THE TRAIL IN MARYLAND IS STEEPED IN HISTORY, PARTICULARLY CONCERNING THE CIVIL WAR ERA.

Maryland

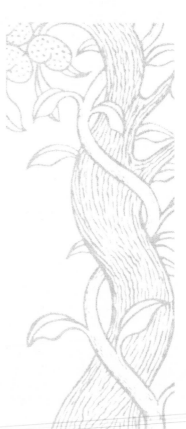

THE APPALACHIAN TRAIL PASSES HIGH ROCK, BUZZARD KNOB, BLACK ROCK CLIFFS, ANNAPOLIS ROCKS, MONUMENT KNOB, WHITE ROCKS, CRAMPTON GAP, AND WEVERTON CLIFFS. OF PARTICULAR HISTORICAL NOTE ARE WASHINGTON MONUMENT STATE PARK (GROUP CAMPING ONLY), TURNERS GAP WITH THE SOUTH MOUNTAIN INN, CRAMPTON GAP WITH GATHLAND STATE PARK (NO CAMPING ALLOWED, AND THE TOWN OF WEVERTON.

BE AWARE THAT MINOR RELOCATIONS ARE PLANNED FOR PORTIONS OF THE TRAIL IN MARYLAND, BUT WILL NOT ADD ANY SIGNIFICANT AMOUNT OF MILEAGE.

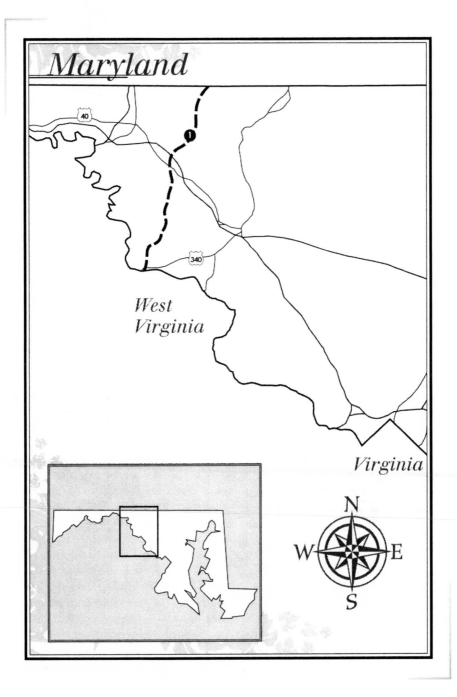

1. Annapolis Rocks to Pen Mar Park

ANNAPOLIS ROCKS
TO PEN MAR PARK

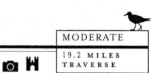

MODERATE

19.2 MILES
TRAVERSE

Numerous vistas and an interesting geological phenomena are the highlights of this overnighter. Annapolis Rocks and Black Rocks Cliff offer spectacular western views of the Maryland countryside, as well as southwestern views of Greenbrier Lake. Raven Rock overlooks Raven Rock Hollow, while High Rock is reached several miles to the north. In between is a side trip to Devils Racecourse, described by some people as being a "river of rock." Although glaciers did not reach this far south, the expansion of freezing water that had seeped into small cracks in the rocks on the hillside caused them to break apart into small pieces and flow into the valley below.

The outing comes to an end as the A.T. descends a boulder field to Pen Mar Park. It appears to be not much more than a community picnic ground today, but the spot was an amazingly popular resort between 1890 and 1920. Seven hotels and close to one hundred guest cottages were located nearby to cater to the daily crowds of five thousand or more that were drawn to an amusement park. Gas rationing during World War II forced the park to close in 1943.

The walking is moderate on this hike, as it takes place along the ridgeline of South Mountain with just a few, short steep ups and downs. Shelters and designated campsites are numerous, so you have a wide choice of where to spend the night.

THE HIKE

From the parking area off US 40, hike the 0.1 mile side trail to the A.T., which you intersect close to the US 40 overpass. Follow a dirt road that climbs into the woods to the right. Turn left in 0.1 mile, and shortly thereafter pass a road leading to a farmhouse on the right.

At mile 0.5, cross a telephone line cut-through, bear right at a fork, and reach the junction with the side trail that leads to Pine Knob Shelter, at 0.6 mile. Water is available from a spring at the shelter.

Continue along the A.T., soon passing another side trail leading to the shelter. Reach a level crest just below Pine Knob at 1.1 miles, pass an old road that intersects the Trail from the right, and pass another old road that intersects the Trail from the left. From here, begin to descend steeply.

At mile 1.9, go left at the fork and reach the side trail to Annapolis Rocks in another 0.4 mile. Take this blue-blazed trail for 0.2 mile to the overhanging rocks that make up this cliff. The views from here are outstanding. This is a popular campsite, and tent platforms have been constructed to ease the impact on the land. Use them and do not create new campsites. A spring is 0.2 mile away via a blue-blazed route.

When you return to the A.T., continue ahead and begin to descend in just over 0.5

mile. At mile 4.1, reach the side trail that leads a little over 100 feet to Black Rock Cliffs. The 180-degree view from this lookout point is equally impressive, and you may want to note the considerable amount of scree at the bottom of the cliff.

Continuing northward on the A.T., cross Black Rock Creek—which may be dry in summer—at 4.6 miles. Walk through the Pogo Memorial Campsite at 4.7 miles. Springs are available near the campsite and via a blue-blazed trail. Beyond this, watch the white blazes carefully as the A.T. makes several turns at old road intersections. The Trail leaves these roads and starts to cross the rocky crest of the mountain at 6.4 miles. Pass by a view to the east at 7.1 miles, and return to old roads at 7.4 miles.

Descend, cross a road at 9.4 miles, and cross a creek 0.1 mile later. Just a few yards beyond, the A.T. swings left, where a blue-blazed side trail leads right 100 feet to an excellent boxed spring. This is the water source for the Ensign Cowall Shelter, whose short side trail you will pass at 9.6 miles.

Continue north on the A.T, cross Foxville Road (Maryland 77), and pass under a power line at 11.8 miles. Descend to pass a spring at 12.1 miles and then ford Little Antietam Creek. Turn left onto Warner Gap Road in 0.2 mile, follow it for only 150 feet, and turn right into the woods to rise over the eastern slope of Buzzard Knob. Cross Little Antietam Creek again at 13 miles and, in another 0.1 mile, cross Maryland 491 diagonally to the right.

Ascend through a forest of deciduous and evergreen trees. The side trail to the right at 13.2 miles will take you about 100 feet to Raven Rock, a prominent cliff with views of the hollow you just walked up from.

Continue on the A.T. and gain the crest of South Mountain. Turn right onto the blue-blazed trail to Devils Racecourse Shelter at 14.1 miles and come to the structure at 14.4 miles. The rocks and boulders of Devils Racecourse fill the valley floor, which is reached via an unmarked trail about 0.1 mile beyond the shelter.

Return to the A.T. and continue northward, passing the highest point of the Trail in Maryland (1,890 feet) on the southern slope of Quirak Mountain at 15.9 miles. A right turn onto the blue-blazed High Rock Loop Trail at 16.6 miles takes you 0.1 mile to High Rock and its sweeping view of the broad Great Valley to the west. This is the same valley that the A.T. parallels and crosses numerous times from southern Virginia all the way to eastern Pennsylvania. Take the other portion of the High Rock Loop Trail back to the A.T and continue northward to begin a steep descent through boulder fields. Be careful and take your time.

After crossing a couple of old roads, you will pass by evidence of former human activity in this area, and turn onto an old railroad bed at 18.9 miles. Soon walk into Pen Mar Park and bring the outing to a close at 19.2 miles.

TRAILHEAD DIRECTIONS

To get to the southern trailhead, take US 40 east from Hagerstown to its first crossing over I-70. The parking lot is immediately to your right after crossing the interstate. A blue-blazed trail leads to the A.T. from the parking area.

Parking for the northern trailhead is in Pen Mar Park or along a residential street of the village of Pen Mar.

THE APPALACHIAN TRAIL IN WEST VIRGINIA IS ABOUT 3 MILES LONG AND IS CENTERED IN THE TOWN OF HARPERS FERRY, WHICH IS HOME TO THE APPALACHIAN TRAIL CONSERVANCY HEADQUARTERS. THE A.T. ALSO PASSES THROUGH WEST VIRGINIA FARTHER SOUTH WHEN THE TRAIL TRAVELS IN SOUTHERN VIRGINIA ALONG THE BORDER OF THE TWO STATES. HERE, THE TRAIL TRAVERSES PETERS MOUNTAIN NORTH OF PEARISBURG, VIRGINIA. THE LONGEST STRETCH OF THE A.T. IS IN

West Virginia
and Virginia

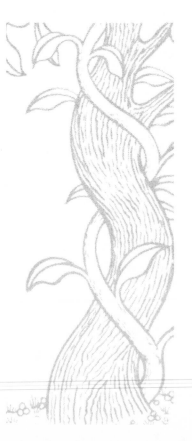

VIRGINIA, WHICH COMPRISES MORE THAN A QUARTER OF THE TRAIL'S LENGTH. FROM THE POTOMAC RIVER NEAR HARPERS FERRY, THE A.T. RIDGE HOPS ALONG THE BLUE RIDGE INTO SHENANDOAH NATIONAL PARK. IT TRAVERSES THE PARK FOR MORE THAN 100 MILES, LEAVING THE PARK BEHIND AT ROCKFISH GAP AND PICKING UP THE BLUE RIDGE PARKWAY, WHICH IT MORE OR LESS PARALLELS FOR 100 MILES UNTIL THE ROANOKE AREA. ALONG THE PARKWAY, IT TRAVERSES HUMPBACK MOUNTAIN, THREE RIDGES, THE PRIEST, SPY ROCK, PUNCHBOWL, AND BLUFF MOUNTAIN, AND DESCENDS TO THE JAMES RIVER. FROM THE JAMES RIVER, THE TRAIL CLIMBS TO APPLE ORCHARD MOUNTAIN, THE HIGHEST POINT ON THE BLUE RIDGE PARKWAY IN VIRGINIA.

In Troutville–Cloverdale, the A.T. heads west toward the border of West Virginia. As it crosses this area, it passes by the remarkable features of Tinker Cliffs and McAfee Knob. The crest of Peters Mountain forms the Virginia–West Virginia border. From here, the A.T. descends to Pearisburg, climbs Angels Rest on Pearis Mountain, and slowly winds its way back toward I-81, though not before crossing I-77 near Bastian, Virginia.

From Atkins, Virginia, the A.T. heads south into the Mount Rogers National Recreation Area, passing through Grayson Highlands State Park and within 0.5 mile of the summit of Mount Rogers, Virginia's highest point. From Mount Rogers, it is less than 30 miles to the Virginia–Tennessee border. In this southern section of Virginia, the Trail traverses White Top Mountain, Buzzard Rock, and Straight Mountain before descending into the hiker-friendly town of Damascus, Virginia. Damascus holds an annual Trail Days festival each May.

About 100 miles of the Appalachian Trail in Virginia pass through Shenandoah National Park. The park is one of the most popular areas to hike along the A.T. Established by President Coolidge in 1926, Shenandoah National Park took ten years to complete. President Roosevelt's Civilian Conservation Corps (CCC) did most of the work. Roosevelt officially dedicated the park in 1936. Skyline Drive was a part of the original concept and took eight years to complete. Beginning construction in 1931, the southern, central and northern sections opened as they were completed (1939, 1934 and 1936, respectively).

Although the A.T. was first constructed in this area in the 1920s and opened in 1929, much of the Trail was relocated as Skyline Drive was built. The CCC was also put to work rebuilding the A.T., and you will note the laborious rockwork that shores up much of the Trail in the park.

The history of the Shenandoah—natural, geologic, and cultural—can and does fill books. For additional information on the park, look for books sold at the park's visitor centers. The flora and fauna of the park is varied

AND INCLUDES EVERYTHING FROM BLACK BEAR AND WHITE-TAILED DEER (THE LATTER, EXTREMELY PREVALENT) TO THE LESS OFTEN SEEN BOBCATS. THE AREAS OF INTENSE DEFOLIATION YOU WILL SEE HAVE BEEN CAUSED BY THE GYPSY MOTH. THE DEER TICK IS ALSO PRESENT IN SHENANDOAH, SO SEARCH YOUR BODY CAREFULLY FOR THIS CARRIER OF LYME DISEASE. AS FOR FLORA, EVERYTHING FROM HEMLOCK-HARDWOOD FORESTS TO BOREAL FORESTS CAN BE FOUND. UNFORTUNATELY, THE HEMLOCKS HAVE BEEN ALMOST TOTALLY DEVASTATED BY THE HEMLOCK WOOLY ADELGID. FLOWERS AND FLOWERING SHRUBS ALSO ABOUND, MAKING THE PARK A FAIRYLAND WALK FROM LATE SPRING THROUGH MID-SUMMER.

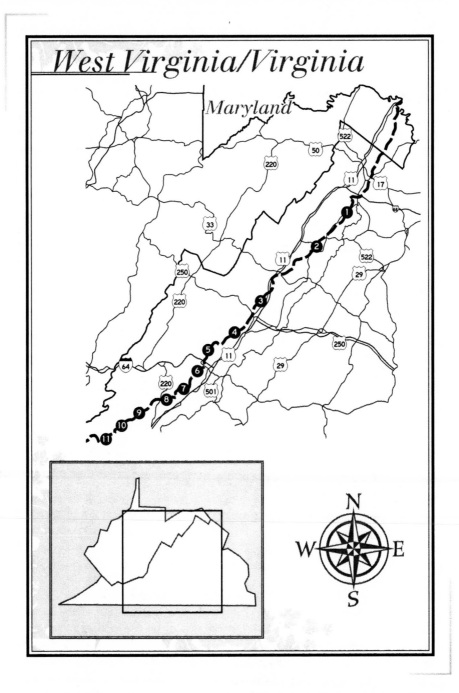

West Virginia/Virginia

Maryland

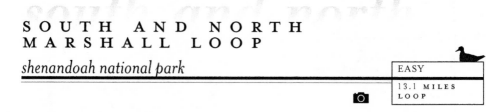

SOUTH AND NORTH MARSHALL LOOP

shenandoah national park

	EASY
	13.1 MILES LOOP

On this loop, you will follow the Mount Marshall, Bluff, and Appalachian Trails as you hike through Shenandoah National Park. There are some moderate climbs along the way, but with only 13 miles to cover in two days, this is an easy weekend hike. This short loop offers several fine views from North and South Marshall Mountains.

North and South Marshall Mountains were once known locally as Bluff Mountain. They were renamed for John Marshall (1755-1835), who served as Chief Justice of the United States for the last 35 years of his life. North and South Marshall Mountains were once owned by the renowned jurist.

THE HIKE

From the parking lot at Jenkins Gap, turn right onto Skyline Drive for 0.1 mile until the junction with the Mount Marshall Trail is reached. Turn left onto this yellow-blazed trail, and soon cross three small streams—Bolton Branch, Waterfall Branch, and Sprucepine Branch—on your way to the junction with the Bluff Trail, 3.6 miles beyond the Jenkins Gap parking lot.

Turn right onto the yellow-blazed Bluff Trail and follow the Trail along the eastern, then southern slopes of North and then South Marshall Mountains, experiencing little change in elevation. At mile 5.8, reach the junction with the blue-blazed Big Devils Stairs Trail. Continue following the yellow-blazed Bluff Trail, and reach a junction with

the Harris Hollow Trail, which shares the same footpath with the Bluff Trail for the next 0.1 mile. As the Harris Hollow Trail turns off to the left, follow the Bluff Trail, which becomes blue blazed.

In 0.1 mile, cross a gravel road leading downhill to Gravel Springs Hut that is for long distance A.T. hikers only. Water is available from a spring at the shelter. Continue following the Bluff Trail for 0.2 mile to the junction with the A.T. Turn right onto the A.T., and hike north for 0.2 mile where it crosses Skyline Drive at milepost 17.7. Continue along the A.T., past where the Browntown Trail meets Skyline Drive. Climb the west slope of Mount Marshall for the next mile. Just before the summit, enjoy fine views from rock outcrops to the left of the Trail.

Reach the summit of South Marshall (elevation 3,212 feet) at mile 8.7, and descend to a gap between South and North Marshall, where you'll cross Skyline Drive at milepost 15.9. Begin climbing North Marshall on switchbacks. During the climb, there are distinct cliffs to the right of the Trail with outstanding views of Skyline Drive and the surrounding mountains and countryside. At mile 9.9, reach the summit of North Marshall (elevation 3,368 feet).

The Trail descends gently from North Marshall and passes a short side trail, which leads to a piped spring in 0.9 mile. In another 0.6 mile, cross Skyline Drive at milepost 14.2 (Hogwallow Gap). Climb from Hogwallow Gap to the top of an unnamed mountain (elevation 2,882 feet), and in 1.7 miles, reach the end of the hike at Jenkins Gap.

TRAILHEAD DIRECTIONS

There is parking for more than a dozen cars at Jenkins Gap. The parking lot is at Skyline Drive milepost 12.3.

STONY MAN AND BIG MEADOWS

shenandoah national park

MODERATE

27 MILES
TRAVERSE

Shenandoah National Park in Virginia is one of the most popular areas to hike along the Appalachian Trail. This traverse takes you south from US 211 at Thornton Gap to Lewis Mountain Campground, passing Marys Rock, Stony Man, Skyland, and Big Meadows.

THE HIKE

Enter the woods on a wide trail from the end of the parking lot, intersect the A.T. in a few feet, and turn left. A break in the vegetation at 0.6 mile provides a view of Thornton Gap, and some of the mountains of the park to the north. At 0.9 mile, cushiony moss growing on boulders along the Trail helps soften the look and feel of a rock field you walk through. The rock walls at 1.2 miles that were built by the Civilian Conservation Corps during the Great Depression to shore up this side hill trail are still performing their duty. Make a right turn onto a side trail at 1.9 miles and ascend 0.1 mile to Marys Rock.

The large outcrop is a favorite bird-watchers' perch to watch the fall hawk migration. A 360-degree view is obtained by scrambling 80 feet to its summit. To the

north is the restaurant and road intersection from which you began the hike. Pass Mountain makes up the ridgeline closest to you, and behind it are the Three Sisters, and Neighbor, Knob, and Hogback Mountains. Scanning to the east you may be able to make out the gorge of Little Devils Stairs between Little Hogback and Mount Marshall. The Piedmont is clearly visible beyond Oventop and Jenkins Mountain. Southward are The Pinnacle and Stony Man, while to the west is Massanutten Mountain rising up to bisect the Shenandoah Valley.

Return to the A.T., following the crest of the ridge with occasional views to the west before descending gradually. In another 0.6 mile, you will reach a sag where Meadow Spring Trail intersects the A.T. from the left. Meadow Spring is 0.25 mile downhill on this side trail. Continue along the narrow crest of the ridge, and enjoy a good view to the west at an outcropping in 0.1 mile.

At mile 3.1, reach another viewpoint, head left, and descend to the base of The Pinnacle. In another 0.3 mile, reach a service road and follow it a short distance to Byrds Nest #3, a day-use shelter with piped water available during warmer months. The service road leads another 0.3 mile to Skyline Drive (milepost 33.9), but the A.T. continues on the ridge, climbs moderately, and reaches a side trail in 0.8 mile.

The side trail leads a short distance to the right to a view north. In another 0.1 mile, you will see the jagged rocks (a short distance to your right) that form the north peak of The Pinnacle. The Trail continues along the crest of the ridge, which has spectacular views of the mountain's sheer western slopes. At mile 4.4, you will reach the highest point of The Pinnacle (elevation 3,730 feet) and begin a descent through mountain laurel. In another 0.7 mile, you will reach the junction with the blue-blazed Leading Ridge Trail, which leads left 0.1 mile to Skyline Drive. The A.T. continues to descend through white pine.

In 0.1 mile, you will pass below the Jewel Hollow Overlook (elevation 3,335 feet) at Skyline Drive milepost 36.4. In another 0.2 mile, you will reach a side trail that heads back a short distance to the Jewel Hollow Overlook. The A.T. continues, climbing moderately along the crest of the ridge, where there are views to the west across Jewel Hollow. Hike 0.1 mile past the side trail to parallel the entrance road to the Pinnacles Picnic Area (milepost 36.7). The A.T. follows the right unpaved fork and skirts the picnic area through laurel.

Pass rest rooms and a water fountain (operational only during warmer months) in another 0.1 mile. Enter the woods, climb briefly, and descend again. At mile 6, pass a notable white pine to your left, and in another 0.1 mile, cross under power lines. Climb to the knob at the head of Nicholson Hollow and in another 0.4 mile turn sharply to the right and descend to a good viewpoint of Nicholson Hollow and Old Rag Mountain.

In 0.1 mile, you will reach an abandoned trail to your right that goes 0.3 mile downhill to a spring near the former site of the Shaver Hollow Shelter. From the side

trail, hike 0.6 mile to the blue-blazed Crusher Ridge Trail, which crosses the A.T. on an old woods road (Sours Lane). At mile 7.3, reach the junction with the blue-blazed Nicholson Hollow Trail. The side trail leads 0.1 mile to Skyline Drive. You will reach another side trail in 0.4 mile that heads left a short distance to the southern end of the Stony Man Mountain Overlook (milepost 38.6) in Hughes River Gap (elevation 3,097 feet). Water and rest rooms are provided at this overlook during the warmer months. From the side trail, the A.T. continues around Nicholson Hollow, parallels Skyline Drive, and ascends.

Reach the side trail to Little Stony Man Parking Area in 0.4 mile. The short side trail heads left to Skyline Drive (milepost 39.1). The A.T. climbs Stony Man moderately on switchbacks and reaches another trail junction at mile 8. Follow the A.T. left at the fork (the right fork, the Passamaquoddy Trail, heads 1.4 miles to Skyland Lodge and is a former A.T. route). Continue another 0.2 mile to the cliffs of Little Stony Man and ascend 0.7 mile to another trail junction.

You could bypass Stony Man, but why would you? It has a grand view and is reached by a 0.4-mile loop. So, turn right and rise to the 4,011-foot summit. Below is Page Valley and the town of Luray, with Massanutten Mountain on the far side. The buildings of Skyland are nearby, and the prominent peak to the south is Hawksbill. The rocky summit you see to the north is Marys Rock. Continue to follow the loop trail, return to the A.T., and resume walking southward. Descend 0.4 mile to the Stony Man Nature Trail Parking Area. The parking area is 0.3 mile to the left of Skyland Lodge and Dining Hall, and 0.1 mile to the right of Skyline Drive (milepost 41.7).

From the parking lot, cross the paved road that leads to Skyland, climb gradually through the woods, and reach the service road to Skyland in 0.2 mile. From here, it is

0.2 mile to the right to Skyland Lodge and Dining Hall. Continue to climb, and soon you will reach an open field with a large green water tank. Descend 0.6 mile to Skyland Road. The road heads left to Skyline Drive and right to Skyland. Continue on the A.T. and hike along the cliffs under Pollock Knob (elevation 3,560 feet) in another 0.3 mile. Pollock Knob and the Passamaquoddy Trail (which means "abounding in Pollock") were named for George Pollock, the founder of Skyland.

The Trail begins to descend via switchbacks at mile 11.6, with great views of Hawksbill Mountain and Ida Valley. Paralleling Skyline Drive, you will pass through a thicket of laurel and reach an open area in 0.5 mile. A side trail to the left heads a short distance uphill to the Timber Hollow Parking Overlook at Skyline Drive (milepost 43.3).

In 0.2 mile, the Trail ascends a small ridge and then descends the western slopes, passing some interesting trees with contorted limbs. An oak, in particular, offers the tired hiker a seat on an extended limb. In 0.7 mile, you will reach a concrete post that marks a side trail that heads right 0.1 mile uphill, just north of Crescent Rock Parking Overlook (milepost 44.4) to good views at Bettys Rock. The Trail continues under the Crescent Rock cliffs. Enjoy great views of Nakedtop and Hawksbill Mountain.

At mile 13.4, you will reach Hawksbill Gap. A side trail turns right downhill and reaches a spring in a short distance. Nearby and to the left is Hawksbill Gap Parking Area on Skyline Drive at milepost 45.6 (elevation 3,361 feet). From the gap, the A.T. climbs up the northern side of Hawksbill Mountain (site of a former peregrine falcon release program) and continues under cliffs. Look behind you for good views of Crescent Rocks, Stony Man, and Old Rag Mountain, and ahead for views of Ida Valley and Luray.

At mile 14.4, you will reach the sag between Hawksbill and Nakedtop; there is a side trail that heads left 0.9 mile to the summit of Hawksbill. The A.T. continues for another 0.3 mile through deep woods before it arrives in an old orchard that is rapidly becoming overrun by other trees. A service road enters from the left from what looks like a grassy meadow. No camping allowed. Continue along the A.T. and within a few feet, reach the side trail (with signpost) that heads right 0.2 mile to Rock Spring Cabin (which may be rented through PATC) and Rock Spring Hut where you may stay overnight without making prior arrangements. From late May through June, A.T. long-distance hikers are likely to fill the shelters in the Shenandoah, but there is still room to camp in the area.

At mile 15.3, you will reach another side trail (with signpost) that heads a short distance uphill to Skyline Drive at Spitler Knoll Parking Overlook (milepost 48.1). The A.T. continues along the slopes before passing a concrete post marking the side trail to the left, which heads uphill 0.25 mile to the north end of Franklin Cliffs Overlook. At mile 16.4, the A.T. passes another side trail, also marked by a post, that heads left 0.3 mile to the south end of Franklin Cliffs Overlook.

At mile 16.6, you will reach the intersection with Red Gate Fire Road in Fishers Gap, formerly Gordonsville Turnpike. The road heads right to Virginia 611 and left to the north end of Fishers Gap Parking Overlook. After passing below the overlook, you will pass another post marking a side trail that heads left a short distance to the Fisher Gap Parking Overlook. In another 0.1 mile, you will pass to the right of a split rock, climb up to a hemlock grove, and cross a small stream twice.

At mile 17.6, locate David Spring a short distance to the right of the A.T. where a trail enters from the left. The A.T. skirts the north edge of Big Meadows Campground. Pass several unmarked trails that lead to the campground. Camping and lodging, food, and water are all available at Big Meadows. Enjoy views along here of Hawksbill Mountain, Stony Man Mountain, Knob Mountain, and Neighbor Mountain.

Cross a small, rocky knob called Monkey Head in 0.3 mile, then skirt the western edge of the ridge, and pass below the amphitheater in Big Meadows in another 0.2 mile. In 0.1 mile, you will pass a concrete post that marks the intersection of the A.T. with the Trail to Lewis Falls 1.2 miles to the right and the Lodge Trail left to the amphitheater parking area. The A.T. continues straight ahead, passing under the sheer cliffs of Blackrock in 0.3 mile. From the rocks there are outstanding views of the Shenandoah Valley, Massanutten Mountain, Great North Mountain, and the Alleghenies rising in the distance.

At mile 18.6, a side trail heads left for 1 mile to a view at Blackrock, and at mile 18.8, another trail leads to Big Meadows Lodge. The A.T. descends the ridge for 0.3 mile to a service road, which leads 0.3 mile left to Skyline Drive (milepost 51.4). The service road reaches Skyline Drive 0.1 mile south of Big Meadows Wayside, where you'll find meals and supplies, and the Harry F. Byrd Sr. Visitor Center. Just past the service road, the A.T. reaches the outlet of the boxed Lewis Spring and continues to descend through the woods for another 0.6 mile before reaching Tanners Ridge Cemetery on the right.

The A.T. continues along a level footpath from here to Milam Gap, just over a mile away. About 0.2 mile after leaving the cemetery, you will pass a spring a short distance to the left of the A.T. Reach Skyline Drive (milepost 52.8) at mile 20.8, south of Milam Gap (elevation 3,257 feet). The A.T. continues east through a field before reaching a concrete post marking the intersection with the Mill Prong Trail to the left. From here, ascend the north ridge of Hazeltop,

bear right at the crest in 0.4 mile and climb moderately to the north end of Hazeltop at mile 22.3.

In another 0.4 mile, you will cross the tree-covered crest of Hazeltop (elevation 3,812 feet). Note the red spruce and balsam on the summit that is marked by a sign. After 0.5 mile, you will reach the intersection of the blue-blazed Laurel Prong Trail, which heads 2.8 miles left to Camp Hoover. In another 0.4 mile, you will reach Bootens Gap (elevation 3,243 feet) and the gate across Conway River Fire Road. Skyline Drive (milepost 55.1) is a short distance to the right. The A.T. descends moderately for 0.2 mile before paralleling Skyline Drive with little change in elevation for the next 0.5 mile.

Begin to climb again along the western slope of Bush Mountain before reaching another trail junction at mile 25. The blue-blazed side trail heads right for 0.1 mile to Bearfence Mountain Parking Area on Skyline Drive (milepost 56.4). For excellent views, follow the side trail left over some rough boulders. You will pass a loop trail over Bearfence Mountain in 0.25 mile, which makes a figure eight with the A.T.

Continue on the A.T. and reach the loop trail noted above in 0.2 mile, where it leaves the A.T. to the left. The loop is only a little longer than the length of the A.T. between the Trail junctions of the loop, and the loop offers outstanding views. But if you continue on the A.T., you will reach the second junction with the loop in another 0.2 mile. From here, the A.T. descends by switchbacks for 0.6 mile to a gap where it intersects the yellow-blazed Slaughter Trail. The side trail heads left 0.1 mile to the access road to Bearfence Mountain Hut, then right a few feet to Skyline Drive (milepost 56.8).

At mile 26.2, another side trail leads left for 0.1 mile to Bearfence Mountain Hut, which is designated for long-distance hikers.

There is a spring a short distance south of the hut that is often dry in the summer. From the hut, the A.T. climbs moderately up Lewis Mountain, leveling off at 3,400 feet. You will pass several paths that lead right to Lewis Mountain Picnic Area and Campground, which is open May through October, but don't leave the A.T. until you reach the post marking the side trail that leads right 100 yards to the campground at mile 26.9. Take this side trail 0.1 mile to the campground and its parking area.

TRAILHEAD DIRECTIONS

The northern trailhead is located next to the Panorama Restaurant in Thornton Gap, at the intersection of US 211 and Skyline Drive (9 miles east of Luray). Leave your car in the parking located on US 211, to access the restaurant and A.T. without having to pass through the park entrance station.

The southern trailhead is in Lewis Mountain Campground, off Skyline Drive at milepost 57.5.

SOUTHERN SHENANDOAH

shenandoah national park

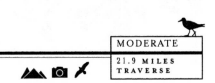

MODERATE

21.9 MILES TRAVERSE

This traverse takes you south from Loft Mountain Campground over the southern Shenandoah to Beagle Gap. In September, Calf Mountain, just north of Beagle Gap, is an excellent site for watching the hawk migrations.

THE HIKE

Begin at Loft Mountain Campground, just past milepost 79 on Skyline Drive. Take the short side trail to the A.T. that begins just south of the Ranger's residence and camp store. The campground has supplies, a laundromat, a phone, and showers. At the junction with the A.T., turn right and begin a moderate ascent of Big Flat Mountain, as you

circle clockwise around the campground near the summit (elevation 3,387 feet). Concrete posts at mile 0.6 and mile 1.1 indicate side trails that lead to the campground. Reach a third concrete post 0.2 mile later that marks the 0.3-mile trail heading to the Loft Mountain Amphitheater. In 0.5 mile, you will reach an outstanding 360-degree view of Rockytop, Brown Mountain, Rocky Mountain, Rocky Mount, and to the far right—east of Skyline Drive—Loft Mountain.

The A.T. descends for another 0.3 mile until it reaches the junction of the Doyles River Trail. A short distance to the right is Skyline Drive (milepost 81.1). Big Run Parking Overlook is a short distance south on Skyline Drive. To the left, it is 0.3 mile to

Doyles River Cabin and spring. The cabin can be rented through the PATC. See the Appendix for more information on how to rent. For the next 0.9 mile, the A.T. parallels Skyline Drive.

At mile 3, the A.T. passes through Doyles River Parking Overlook (milepost 81.9 on Skyline Drive). Follow the ledges (with good winter views) and cross to the right of Skyline Drive (milepost 82.2). From Skyline Drive, enjoy a good view of Cedar and Trayfoot Mountains. At mile 3.7, you will reach the intersection of the Big Run Loop Trail and then begin a moderate descent. In another 0.6 mile, you will arrive at the concrete post marking the junction with the Madison Run Fire Road a short distance to the right of Skyline Drive (milepost 82.9). This is Browns Gap (elevation 2,599 feet), which was used by General Stonewall Jackson during the Civil War. The A.T. crosses Skyline Drive diagonally to the left and begins to ascend. At mile 4.7, the A.T. skirts to the east of Dundo Campground (a developed area at milepost 83.7) for the next 0.2 mile. Water is available at Dundo from May through October.

When a trail heads right to the Dundo Campground Area, follow the A.T. left and reach the junction with the Jones Run Trail in 0.6 mile. Jones Run Parking Area is a short distance to the right. The A.T. continues ahead, soon passing through an old apple orchard and then crossing Skyline Drive (milepost 84.3) at mile 5.8. The Trail begins a moderate climb for 0.6 mile until the A.T. and the Trayfoot Mountain Trail come within a few feet of each other but do not cross. The trails parallel each other for about 0.1 mile before the A.T. turns right and circles the sides of Blackrock (elevation 3,092 feet) with its tumbled, lichen-covered boulders.

At mile 6.8, you will reach the blue-blazed Blackrock Spur Trail, which heads right along the ridge to Trayfoot Mountain.

In another 0.1 mile, the A.T. crosses Trayfoot Mountain Trail and begins a descent to Blackrock Gap. At mile 7.4, you will reach the side trail to Blackrock Hut. It's only 0.2 mile away in a deep ravine with a spring near the front of the hut, where you can stay overnight. From late May through June, A.T. long distance hikers are likely to fill the shelters in the Shenandoah, but there is still room to camp in the area.

The A.T. continues ahead and crosses an old road a short distance later. It then parallels the road for 0.2 mile, then joins it and follows the road to its junction with Skyline Drive (milepost 87.2). Cross the Drive, continue along its east side for 0.2 mile, and reach Moormans River Fire Road (yellow blazes) at Blackrock Gap (milepost 87.4). The fire road heads 9.4 miles to Jarman Gap. The A.T. ascends a small knob and then descends to a sag at mile 9.2, where Skyline Drive is a short distance to the right. From here, the Trail ascends a second small knob.

At mile 9.9, the Trail crosses Skyline Drive (milepost 88.9) in a sag and ascends again, reaching the intersection with the blue-blazed Riprap Trail in 0.7 mile at the summit of a knob (elevation 2,988 feet). From here, descend steeply, and in 0.4 mile, reach a graded trail that heads left to the Riprap Parking Area on Skyline Drive (milepost 90). Descend steeply for another 0.1 mile and then descend more gradually. Follow a path that rolls gently up and down for 2 miles. Keep an eye out for the Catawba rhododendrons in this section.

You will reach the junction of the Wildcat Ridge Trail at mile 13.7. The Wildcat Ridge Parking Area on Skyline Drive (milepost 92.1) is a short distance to the left. The A.T. climbs moderately, crosses Skyline Drive (milepost 92.4) in 0.3 mile, then continues to ascend, reaching a summit (elevation 3,080 feet) in 0.5 mile. The Trail then descends to a slight sag before regaining the lost elevation, then descending steeply again toward Turk Gap.

At mile 16, the A.T. reaches a concrete post marking the beginning of the Turk Branch Trail, which leaves the A.T. to the left. The A.T. crosses Skyline Drive at Turk Gap (milepost 94.1) and joins the Turk Mountain Trail for 0.2 mile before the Turk Mountain Trail leaves the A.T. to the right. Continue ahead on the A.T., reaching the crest of the ridge a short distance later, and begin a long, moderate descent.

At mile 17.6, in a deep sag at the northern edge of the Sawmill Run Parking Overlook, the A.T. crosses Skyline Drive (milepost 95.3) and begins to ascend. While ascending, look over your shoulder for views of Turk Mountain, Sawmill Ridge, and the city of Waynesboro. Hike 0.5 mile to the summit of an unnamed hill (elevation 2,453 feet), and as the Trail begins to descend, enjoy views to the east of Bucks Elbow Mountain. In another 0.4 mile, cross a grass-covered pipe line cut-through and continue to descend.

You will reach the South Fork of Moormans River 0.3 mile later, which here is just a small creek. Follow the west bank of the creek to its source, and continue along the A.T. another 0.2 mile to the Moormans River Fire Road. The road heads left 0.1 mile to Skyline Drive at Jarman Gap (milepost 96.8). A short distance later, after crossing the road, you will pass a spring to your left and begin to ascend.

At mile 19.4 you will reach the Bucks Elbow Mountain Fire Road, which is a short distance east of Skyline Drive (milepost 96.9), and begin to climb toward the south. In another 0.4 mile, you will pass a spring to your left, and 0.2 mile later, you will cross a power line cut-through. At mile 20, you will reach a side trail that heads right 0.2 mile to a spring, and another 0.1 mile to Calf Mountain Shelter. This is a shelter, not a hut, and can be used by short-distance hikers as well as long-distance hikers.

Hike 0.3 mile to an open area, where the Trail follows a pasture road through grass and staghorn sumac, and reach the summit of Calf Mountain (elevation 2,974 feet) in another 0.3 mile. In the fall, this is an excellent site for watching the hawk migrations. The A.T. continues along the ridge before descending through pines and crossing a stone fence. At mile 21.6, the A.T. passes to the left of Little Calf Mountain and descends 0.3 mile to Beagle Gap at Skyline Drive (milepost 99.5).

TRAILHEAD DIRECTIONS

Loft Mountain Campground is between mileposts 79 and 80 on Skyline Drive. Parking is available in the campground close to the store. Parking is available for the southern end of the hike in a small pullout in Beagle Gap, milepost 99.5 on Skyline Drive.

MILL CREEK AND
HUMPBACK MOUNTAIN

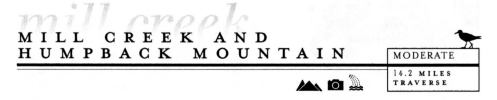

MODERATE

14.2 MILES
TRAVERSE

This initial section of the Appalachian Trail to parallel the Blue Ridge Parkway is quite enjoyable as it contours around the mountainsides and past several small water runs. The walking is made even more pleasurable by the fact that the route uses old roadways that were once important transportation links for the inhabitants of the central Blue Ridge Mountains. When not following these roadbeds, you will be on superbly constructed pathways built by volunteers of the Old Dominion Appalachian Trail Club and ATC's Konnarock Crew. In addition, the isolation in Mill Creek Valley allows you to forget you are so close to the parkway.

Rising from the creek, the A.T. passes the short side trail to Humpback Rocks—with its superb vista—and goes over the summit of Humpback Mountain for views to the east and west.

Camping is only permitted at the Wolfe Shelter, so your first day will be rather short, with the second day being a hike of just under ten miles.

THE HIKE

At the very start of the Blue Ridge Parkway in Rockfish Gap, the A.T. drops to the east of the scenic highway and follows the minor downs and ups of an old woods road. As you level out in an area of large grapevines at 1.3 miles, the A.T leaves the roadbed and follows a footpath to the right, soon merging

onto another old road. However, just 0.3 mile later, the Trail veers left onto a wide and well-built footpath, soon crossing a creek valley and ascending to a long stretch of minor ups and downs.

At 3.4 miles you will pass through an area that bears evidence of previous mountain farm use and ascend on an old woods road. In 0.2 mile, the A.T. turns left off the road and descends via switchbacks. At 5 miles, arrive at your destination for the night, the Paul C. Wolfe Shelter. Enjoy the peace and quiet of this isolated mountain valley, and maybe head downstream about 100 feet to take a swim in the base of a waterfall in Mill Creek.

Cross the creek and rise, again on well-constructed switchbacks. Pass by a view of Rockfish Valley, Rockfish Gap, and the mountains in the southern part of Shenandoah National Park at 5.7 miles. In 0.3 mile, the A.T. swings left onto an old road, while the blue-blazed Dobie Mountain Trail (an old A.T. route) goes off to the right. Stay left again in another 0.6 mile when a blue-blazed trail goes off to the right (and reaches Humpback Gap parking area in 1 mile).

A side trail to the left at 6.8 miles leads 0.2 mile to a view of Glass Hollow. Continue on the A.T., and at 7.6 miles, swing left onto an old woods road (Howardsville Turnpike), which was a major trade road that connected the Rockfish and Shenandoah Valleys in the 1800s. A right turn would take you to the parking area in 0.2 mile. Soon, ascend switchbacks to pass by Bear Spring at mile 9 and a second spring at 9.8 miles.

Turn right onto the side trail at 10.6 miles and follow it for 0.2 mile to another right turn to reach Humpback Rocks at 10.9 miles for grand views of Back Creek Valley and Pine Ridge. Return to the A.T., continue south and cross the summit of Humpback Mountain at 12.2 miles. Rock outcroppings permit views of Rockfish Gap and the mountains of Shenandoah National Park to the north, Shenandoah Valley to the west, and Rockfish Valley to the east.

At 13.3 miles is a view of Wintergreen Resort to the south. It is time to leave the A.T. at 13.9 miles and follow the blue-blazed trail to the right for 0.3 mile to the Humpback Rocks Picnic Area and the end of the hike.

TRAILHEAD DIRECTIONS

The northern trailhead is on the Blue Ridge Parkway where it crosses Interstate 64 and US 250 in Rockfish Gap. This point is 4 miles east of Waynesboro, Virginia, by way of US 250, or 21 miles west of Charlottesville, Virginia, via I-64 and then US 250.

The hike ends in the Humpback Rocks Picnic Area at Blue Ridge Parkway milepost 8.5. The trailhead is at the rear of the picnic area.

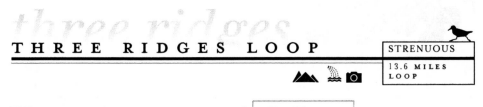

THREE RIDGES LOOP

STRENUOUS

13.6 MILES
LOOP

You will follow the A.T. and Mau-Har Trail on this short overnight hike. There are several fine viewpoints on the A.T. portion of this hike, which climbs to the summit of Three Ridges. The Mau-Har Trail boasts a 40-foot waterfall and creates an easier descent back to the Tye River. Also of note is the 100-foot-long suspension bridge over the Tye River, which was built by the U.S. Forest Service.

All in all, this is an outstanding weekend hike, but it is not to be underestimated. Although the hike is less than 14 miles long, there is a 3,000-foot change in elevation from the Tye River (elevation 920 feet) to the summit of Three Ridges (elevation 3,970 feet) and most of the change comes in 3 miles of climbing.

THE HIKE

From Virginia 56, follow the A.T. north and descend gradually. In 0.1 mile, cross the 100-foot suspension bridge over the Tye River. The A.T. begins climbing on switchbacks, and in 1.7 miles, reaches the junction with the Mau-Har Trail. Continue following the A.T. and cross Harper Creek in 0.8 mile. In another 0.1 mile, a blue-blazed side trail leads to Harpers Creek Shelter. Water is available from the creek.

The climb gets steeper beyond the side trail to the shelter. In 1.6 miles, enjoy a view of The Priest, and in another 0.1 mile, cross the lowest of the ridges that make up the mountain. Beyond the crest of that ridge, hike 0.3 mile to Chimney Rock, a boulder pile to the left of the A.T. Just beyond the boulders, at mile 4.6, pass a viewpoint on the right side of the Trail and then cross the crest of the second ridge.

The last of the three ridges is the toughest climb. After 1.4 miles, the climb eases, and in another 0.3 mile, at mile 6.3, reach the wooded summit of Three Ridges (elevation 3,970 feet). Hike a moderate 0.5 mile, descending to Hanging Rock, which provides views of The Priest and the valley below. Continue descending Three Ridges, and in 0.5 mile, begin climbing again. In 1.1 mile, reach the summit of Bee Mountain (elevation 3,034 feet) and descend. In another 0.4 mile, turn left onto the blue-blazed trail that leads 0.1 to Maupin Field Shelter. This is a good point to break up the hike. Although the first day is long and

hard, it allows for a shorter second day with time to enjoy the waterfall and get home for dinner.

Follow the Mau-Har Trail behind the shelter and, in 1.5 miles, reach the 40-foot falls on Campbell Creek, the highlight of this trail. Continue following the Mau-Har Trail, and in another 1.5 miles reach the junction with the A.T. Turn right on the A.T. and hike south 1.7 miles to the suspension bridge over the Tye River. From there it is a short climb to Virginia 56, the end of this hike.

TRAILHEAD DIRECTIONS

The A.T. crosses VA 56 about 1.4 miles west of Tyro, Virginia, and 11.3 miles east of the Blue Ridge Parkway.

BALD KNOB TO THE PRIEST

MODERATE

25.7 MILES
TRAVERSE

At the beginning of this hike, you climb to the wooded summit of Bald Knob. The name may seem inappropriate, but the knob was once a cleared mountain. Summertime hikers might think that the rest of the hike will be through a tunnel of green, but as you will soon see, this overnight hike has a lot of magnificent views to offer. As you climb across the grassy summits of Cold Mountain and Tar Jacket Ridge, you are afforded spectacular panoramic views. Both highpoints were once used as pasture land; the cleared highlands are the result of years of cattle grazing. Cold Mountain and Tar Jacket Ridge are now mowed by members of

the Natural Bridge Appalachian Trail Club with funding from the Appalachian Trail Conservancy and in partnership with the US Forest Service to maintain both as balds.

This hike will also take you to Spy Rock; the name dates back to its use as a Confederate lookout point in the Civil War. The last mountain you will climb is The Priest; the wooded summit towers over the Tye River Valley. The descent down sometimes steep switchbacks takes you from The Priest to the highway nearly 3,000 feet below.

This hike is described as moderate, but be prepared for a couple of short strenuous sections at each end of the hike.

NOTE: A minor reroute was under construction as this book went to press, but the overall mileage of this hike will not increase greatly.

THE HIKE

From US 60, follow the A.T. north and begin climbing Bald Knob. In 2.8 miles, reach the tree-covered summit of Bald Knob (elevation 4,059 feet). Descend from the Knob, and in 1 mile, pass a 0.6-mile side trail on the right to Cow Camp Gap Shelter. Water is available from a nearby spring.

Following the A.T. north, climb 1 mile, and walk onto the grassy crest of Cold Mountain. Hike another 0.2 mile to the rocks at the summit of Cold Mountain (elevation 4,022 feet). From Cold Mountain, enjoy a tremendous panorama of the surrounding mountains including a view of the remainder of your hike. In the foreground to the northeast, you can see the grassy top of Tar Jacket Ridge. Farther away and a bit to the east, view the peaks of the Religious Range. The closest mountain is the Cardinal, and in the distance, you can see Little Priest and The Priest.

Descend Cold Mountain on the A.T., reach USFS 48 in Hog Camp Gap at mile 6.3, and in 0.9 mile, reach a high point along Tar Jacket Ridge (elevation 3,847 feet). Like Cold Mountain, the grassy ridge offers a noteworthy panoramic view. Continue north, descend Tar Jacket Ridge, and reach USFS 63 in Salt Log Gap at mile 8.5.

The Trail climbs out of Salt Log Gap, crossing USFS 246 in 1.2 miles. Reach USFS 1176A, locally known as Greasy Spring Road, 0.5 mile beyond Salt Log Gap. Continue north on the A.T. and climb to Wolf Rocks Overlook in another 1 mile. Rocky Mountain is the peak to the southwest with antennas on top. To the northeast, view The Priest. After a short descent, the Trail is evenly graded along sidehill until the 0.1-mile side trail to the Seeley-Woodworth Shelter at mile 14. Camping here breaks the hike up into two roughly equal sections. Water is available from a spring near the shelter.

After passing the side trail to the shelter, the Trail passes through an open meadow with views of Spy Rock and The Priest during the 2.3 miles to Virginia 690 (locally known as Fish Hatchery Road). Beyond the road, climb, somewhat steeply, for 0.5 mile to the junction with the side trail leading 0.1 mile to Spy Rock. Spy Rock is the best viewpoint on this hike, and is well worth the short, but steep and rocky climb; the dome-shaped Spy Rock offers a spectacular view of the entire Religious Range as well as other surrounding peaks.

In 0.3 mile, cross the summit of Maintop Mountain (elevation 4,040 feet). Descend Maintop for the next 2.2 miles and reach the dirt Cash Hollow Road at mile 19.2. The Trail climbs over an unnamed high point and descends to Virginia 826 (locally known as Crabtree Farm Road) in 0.8 mile. In 0.7 mile, during the climb up The Priest, reach the junction with an unblazed trail that leads 1.5 miles to Little Priest. Continue to follow the A.T. for 0.2 mile to the side trail leading 0.1 mile to The Priest Shelter. Water is available from a nearby spring. From the shelter side trail, pass by three trails to the left that lead to limited views. Take the fourth route to the left (which is 0.4 mile from from the shelter side trail) for 150 feet for views of Pinnacle Rock ahead, Spy Rock and Main Top to the left, and Humpback and Three Ridges to the right. Return to the A.T. and attain the wooded summit of The Priest (elevation 4,063 feet) in 0.1 mile. Descend The Priest on switchbacks, cross Cripple Creek in 3 miles, and descend another 1.3 miles to Virginia 56, the end of the hike.

The southern end of this hike is at US 60, which the A.T. crosses 9.3 miles east of US 501 in Buena Vista, Virginia. The northern end of the hike is at the Tye River on VA 56. This trailhead is 11.3 miles east of the Blue Ridge Parkway and 1.4 miles west of Tyro, Virginia.

THUNDER HILL TO JENNINGS CREEK

MODERATE

15.4 MILES
TRAVERSE

After beginning with an Olympian view of the Great Valley of Virginia, this hike follow a superb relocation by volunteers of the Natural Bridge Appalachian Trail Club and ATC's Konnarock Crew that brought the Trail back to its original 1930s location. Rising on 110 rock steps, the Trail winds in and around several interesting rock formations, including The Guillotine, a large boulder that hangs over the Trail, trapped in a cleft of another rock. It then goes over the summit of Apple Orchard Mountain, which has another nice view and a large Federal Aviation Administration air-traffic radar dome antenna. The antenna is all that remains of the Bedford Air Force Base, which operated on the summit from 1954 to 1974. As many as 120 airmen were stationed on the mountain during those 20 years.

It is primarily a downhill journey from here, passing by a few more views, the multi-leveled Bryant Ridge Shelter, and ending next to a wonderful swimming hole at Jennings Creek.

THE HIKE

Take the Thunder Ridge Loop Trail from the upper end of the parking lot and intersect the A.T. in 50 yards. Stay to the left and come to a sweeping view of the Great Valley of Virginia, bisected by the James River and framed by the Allegheny Mountains to the west. The loop trail leaves the A.T. in another 0.1 mile; stay right, cross the Blue Ridge Parkway in an additional 0.3 mile, and pass blue-blazed Hunting Creek Trail in 0.1 mile. Continue on the A.T, gradually rising and then gradually descending to the Thunder Hill Shelter at 1.4 miles. Water is from a spring that may be dry in late summer.

Cross the parkway at 1.7 miles, ascend, pass through The Guillotine at 2.3 miles, and break out of the woods to rise to the summit of Apple Orchard Mountain at 2.6 miles. Views of mountain peaks more than 40 miles away are visible from rocks just a few feet off the Trail to the left. Descend onto the wooded slope of Apple Orchard Mountain, dotted with trillium and other wildflowers in the spring. Cross USFS 812 (Parkers Gap Road) at 4 miles and soon cross blue-blazed Apple Orchard Falls Trail, which goes right 1 mile to the falls and left 0.2 mile to Sunset Field Overlook at Blue Ridge Parkway milepost 78.4.

Continue on the A.T., reach the ridge-line at 4.7 miles, and descend to pass by blue-blazed Cornelius Creek National Recreation Trail at 5.2 miles. A side trail at 5.8 miles goes 200 feet to Black Rocks and a view of Headforemost Mountain, Floyd Mountain, Pine Ridge, and other ridgelines to the west.

After crossing two branches of Cornelius Creek along the A.T., a side trail to the left at 6.7 miles goes 0.1 mile to Cornelius Creek Shelter. From a view back to the FAA antenna atop Apple Orchard Mountain at 7.8 miles, the A.T. begins a long descent, before rising and falling a number of times. The blue-blazed trail at 11.5 miles goes left 0.5 mile to Virginia 714. Pass by Bryant Ridge Shelter at 11.6 miles and soon cross Hamps Branch. Another blue-blazed trail, this one at 13.2 miles, goes left for 0.8 mile to VA 714. Rise to the ridgeline in 0.6

mile and, after 0.3 mile, descend to Virginia 614 at 15.4 miles. Jennings Creek, with an appealing swimming hole, is located next to the trailhead parking area.

TRAILHEAD DIRECTIONS

The northern trailhead is in the Thunder Ridge Overlook parking area at Blue Ridge Parkway milepost 74.7. Leave your car at the upper end of the lot.

The southern trailhead is on Virginia 614, 4.6 miles north of Arcadia, Virginia. It may be reached from the Blue Ridge Parkway at milepost 89.1 in Powells Gap by following Virginia 618, then VA 614 for a total of 5.8 miles to the A.T. crossing of Jennings Creek on Panther Ford Bridge.

DRAGON'S TOOTH, MCAFEE KNOB, AND TINKER CLIFFS

STRENUOUS

23.6 MILES TRAVERSE

On one of her three thru-hikes of the A.T., Laurie "The Umbrella Lady" Adkins dubbed Dragon's Tooth, McAfee Knob, and Tinker Cliffs as Virginia's Triple Crown—of viewpoints, that is. Many locals invest the time of several day hikes in order to reach these points, but on just a single overnight journey you can visit all three, considered by many to be some of the best vistas within the Old Dominion. Dragon's Tooth is a monolithic formation rising vertically above the tree tops, McAfee Knob juts horizontally into space, and Tinker Cliffs is a half-mile of sheer rock walls running along the crest of a ridge.

A moderately strenuous, but not entirely difficult hike, this outing makes use of the Appalachian Trail and two side routes. Water sources are few and far between, so be sure to fill up whenever you encounter one. Although you can make use of trail-side shelters, it would still be a wise idea to carry a tent, as the shelters often fill up quickly on the weekends.

THE HIKE

Enter the woods on the blue-blazed Dragon's Tooth Trail, cross a couple of footbridges, rock hop a stream and come to a junction at

0.2 mile. The Boy Scout Trail goes left; you need to turn to the right, beginning your ascent along a water drainage route. This portion of the pathway was slightly relocated in the late 1990s, avoiding some of the more wet and eroded areas, but adding about 0.2 mile to the overall length of the Trail. As you climb, the pine trees become less prevalent and are replaced by hardwoods, such as oak and maple.

A series of switchbacks delivers you to the intersection with the A.T. in Lost Spectacles Gap at 1.7 miles. Tom Campbell, a member of the Roanoke Appalachian Trail Club (RATC), who was a pioneer in relocating the A.T. west of the Blue Ridge in the 1950s, gave this place its name after misplacing his glasses here during a scouting and work hike.

The initial, easy portion of your outing is over once you turn right onto the A.T. and start the climb across the eastern side of Cove Mountain. Occasional views of the Catawba Valley to the east may distract you from watching where you should place your feet along this rocky route. Volunteers with the Appalachian Trail Conservancy and RATC have devoted many hours working on this route, moving huge boulders, constructing rock steps, and defining the correct route. However, the steep and craggy terrain insures that this will continue to be a rugged hike.

After negotiating the rocks and boulders, reach the crest of Cove Mountain (3,020 feet) at 2.7 miles, take your leave of the A.T., and turn left onto the blue-blazed pathway leading just a few hundred feet to the Dragon's Tooth. Although you can obtain the same grand view of Catawba Valley, McAfee Knob, Tinker Mountain, and the Peaks of Otter from its lower portions, those of you who are adventurous can climb to the tooth's crown via a crack. Use caution: a number of people have fallen and sustained serious injuries.

Retrace your steps back down to Lost Spectacles Gap at 3.7 miles, bypass the blue-blazed Dragon's Tooth Trail, and ascend along the white-blazed A.T. Devil's Seat, a rocky outcrop to the right at 3.9 miles, grants an additional view of the Catawba Valley. The deep cleft along Sawtooth Ridge that you see almost directly in front of you is Beckner Gap, which you will be walking next to in just a few more miles.

The rocky ridgeline descends and begins to narrow at 4 miles, where Viewpoint Rock looks onto VA 311 snaking its way between Cove and North Mountains. The ridge crest becomes even narrower where it courses its way through the sandstone rocks of Rawies Rest at 4.3 miles. More than 400 million years old, the boulders are believed to have been formed during momentous volcanic eruptions.

Continue with the gradual descent, obtaining occasional vistas and coming to an intersection at 4.9 miles. The blue-blazed Boy Scout Trail heads off to the left; you want to keep right along the A.T., descend into a stand of pines, and cross VA 624 at 5.3 miles. (Camping is permitted only at designated sites and shelters from here to the end of the hike. Please observe this rule and refrain from using any unauthorized sites you may find along the way. Usage is heavy along this section of the A.T. and authorities are trying to prevent any additional erosion and destruction of vegetation.)

Immediately begin to rise on a switchbacked route which, in early spring, passes through a veritable garden of wildflowers. Columbine, gaywings, and trout lily grow so abundantly that many of them spring up from the soil in the middle of the Trail. Upon obtaining the top of Sandstone Ridge at 5.8 miles, descend into a young forest on the mountain's eastern face. This land was primarily open fields when the A.T. was relocated onto it in the 1980s, but is now on its way to becoming a mature forest. Join an old woods road and use a wooden bridge at 6.2 miles to step over a stream. Stop for just a moment and appreciate your surroundings. Because so few people, other than thruhikers, traverse this section of the A.T., this fetchingly serene, narrow valley is a hidden gem—one which you have now been permitted to experience.

Break out into an open cattle pasture at 6.5 miles, being mindful of where you step. Watch for the white blazes painted upon posts and fencelines to direct you through the field, over a couple of stiles, and onto a crossing of VA 785 at 6.8 miles. Step over another stile on the opposite side of VA 785, walk through a meadow, cross a footbridge over Catawba Creek at 6.9 miles, and make use of yet another stile a few feet later. After negotiating an additional stile at 7.1 miles, cross a small stream and ascend into an open meadow with Beckner Gap rising to your right. It might be time to take another break just before entering the woods at 7.3 miles. Turn around to let your eyes gaze across everything you have traversed so far—the two meadows, Sandstone Ridge, the eastern flank of Cove Mountain and, towering above it all, the distinct, uplifted rock of Dragon's Tooth.

Enter the woods, continue to rise toward the ridgeline via switchbacks lined by trout lily, and cross another stile at 7.5 miles. Amidst white and Virginia pine, attain the crest of Sawtooth Ridge at 7.8 miles and begin to traverse the undulations of this terrain, which its name so aptly describes. Although there are many ups and downs for the next several miles, they rarely involve much more than 100 feet of elevation change. As you progress from one knoll to the next, thank the volunteers of the RATC who spent many hours digging sidehill trail to eliminate a large percentage of the formerly steep ascents and descents.

Be on the lookout for jack-in-the-pulpit all along this route, but especially in the low point you walk into at 9.1 miles. Once you begin the final downhill on Sawtooth Ridge, there will be an excellent view of Mason Cove and Fort Lewis Mountain from an outcropping to the right at 10.8 miles. The traffic zooms by at a high rate of speed, so use caution crossing VA 311 at 11.1 miles.

By way of a couple of switchbacks, reach the ridgeline of Catawba Mountain at 11.3 miles and continue to ascend along its rocky crest. Upon reaching a trailhead bulletin board at 11.4 miles, with a nice view of Mason Cove and Fort Lewis Mountain on the right, the route becomes sidehill trail, running a few hundred feet below the main ridgeline. Serviceberry, iris, Bowman's root, fire pink, Indian pipe, chickweed, buttercup, and violets are just a few of the scores of plants which make this section of the A.T. a particular favorite of wildflower disciples.

An outhouse and Johns Spring Shelter are just to the right of the Trail at 12.1 miles. A series of ups and downs brings the Trail onto a descending woods road at 13 miles, which, in turn, goes by a developed spring just a few hundred feet later. Cross a small stream and come to Catawba Mountain Shelter, at 13.1 miles. A designated campsite is just a few hundred feet beyond the shelter.

Cross a dirt fire road within 0.3 mile of leaving the shelter, pass through thick laurel growth and head toward McAfee Knob. After making a slight dip, the pathway resumes the climb and turns left onto a woods road at 14.4 miles. Local old timers reminisce about driving their cars to the top of McAfee Knob, one of their favorite "romancing" spots.

The Trail splits at 14.5 miles, and to get the most enjoyment from McAfee Knob, take the blue-blazed side trail to the left. Within 100 feet you will break out of the woods and come to what many A.T. thruhikers believe to be the best view in all of

Virginia. To the west are the Catawba Valley, North Mountain, and distant Potts Mountain. Directly in front is the ridgeline you will be walking upon to Tinker Cliffs, and to the northeast you can trace the route of the Appalachian Trail all of the way to the Peaks of Otter and Apple Orchard Mountain, nearly 60 miles away. On very clear days you can make out the bulk of House Mountain almost due north.

Walk by The Anvil (it juts out into space) along the rock outcropping and come to its end with a view of the city of Roanoke nestled within the Great Valley of Virginia. Rejoin the A.T. and continue northward by descending into the Devils Kitchen, a jumble of cracked and broken giant sandstone formations.

Lousewort grows in abundance along the switchbacks you use to descend the north side of the knob. The Pig Farm Campsite is to the right of the Trail at 15.2 miles. Swine were raised near here until as late as 1982. In fact, much of the land you have walked upon on Catawba Mountain was open farmland, and only began to grow back to forest once it was purchased for the A.T.

The Campbell Shelter is to the right of the Trail in another 0.1 mile, while lily of the valley and spiderworts line the pathway as you continue northward. Turn left onto a woods road at 16 miles, only to leave it at 16.7 miles and ascend to the left. Pass between two large rocks, known as Snack Bar Rock, at 17 miles, and walk beside an overhanging slab—Rock Haven—at 17.3 miles. The outcropping at 17.6 miles provides the excuse needed to take a rest break and enjoy the views of Carvin's Cove (a water supply for Roanoke), Tinker Mountain, Peaks of Otter, and Apple Orchard Mountain. Turn your gaze back toward the way you came and look up to McAfee Knob.

Descending into Brickey Gap at 18.2 miles, a blue blaze trail leads right to Lam-

berts Meadow; you want to stay on the A.T. and begin the final climb to Tinker Cliffs. Fringe tree, one of the last trees to bear flowers and leaves late in spring, occupies much of the understory along this section of the hike. Its genus name, *chioanthus*, means "snow flower" and justly describes its blossoms.

Walk onto the southern end of Tinker Cliffs at 19.5 miles, the last of the Triple Crown views. Stretching for half a mile, the rock cliffs overlook the Catawba Valley, Gravelly Ridge, and North Mountain. Once again, you can gaze upon McAfee Knob to the south. Use caution, especially if it has been raining or snowing, as you proceed along the narrow edge, which has bluets and stonecrop growing out of its small nooks and cracks.

Upon reaching the north end of the cliffs at 20 miles, make a quick descent on switchbacks, watching for the yellowish-brown spikes of squawroot, and coming to yellow-blazed Andy Layne Trail in Scorched Earth Gap at 20.5 miles. (Lamberts Meadow Shelter is another 0.7 mile north on the A.T.) Tom Campbell is also credited with providing the name of this spot. According to the RATC lore, he and fellow hikers were on another scouting trip and had just climbed Tinker Mountain, via what is now the Andy Layne Trail. A female participant, known to be quite religious, surprised everyone with her anger at the steepness of the route. She let loose such a volatile succession of expletives that Campbell said she had "scorched the earth."

Descend westward along the Andy Layne Trail, now not quite as steep as it once was, thanks to a relocation that was dedicated in 2001. The pathway is named in memory of one of the hardest working, and jovial, volunteer trail workers in the history of the Appalachian Trail Conservancy. The route at first descends along a narrow waterway and then down the crest of a spur ridge to cross Catawba Creek on a footbridge at 22.7 miles. Walk downstream, with black-eyed Susans dotting the meadow from mid-summer to late fall.

Use the bridge over Little Catawba Creek at 23 miles and pass through more cattle pastures before traversing a young forest to arrive at VA 779 at 23.6 miles.

TRAILHEAD DIRECTIONS

For the northern trailhead, take I-81 Exit 150 a few miles north of Roanoke, drive 1.7 miles on US 220, turn left onto VA 779 (Catawba Road), and pull into the unmarked parking lot on the left in another 8.5 miles. The southern trailhead may be reached by taking I-81 Exit 141 near Roanoke and driving VA 419 to the north for less than 0.5 mile. Make a right turn at the stoplight and follow VA 311 north for 10.5 miles. The parking lot for the Dragon's Tooth Trail is clearly marked on the left side of the road.

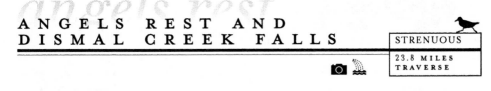

ANGELS REST AND DISMAL CREEK FALLS

STRENUOUS

23.8 MILES TRAVERSE

Several excellent views are your reward for climbing close to 1,500 feet from the New River Valley to the top of Pearis Mountain. Long, gradually rising switchbacks, constructed by volunteers of the Roanoke Appalachian Trail Club, ease the huff-and-puff factor. Once on top, the walking is easy as you follow the crest of Pearisburg Mountain for many miles. A couple of more views and a quick descent bring you to Dismal Creek Falls, a great trout fishing and swimming stream.

The hike is a good choice from early spring when wildflowers are abundant, into mid-June when the rhododendron bushes burst forth with thousand of blossoms, and through mid-September when the waters of Dismal Creek have warmed enough to let you swim without having chattering teeth.

THE HIKE

Ascend the A.T. to the south. At 0.2 mile, pass a spring that may not be running in dry weather. Within a mixed hardwood forest, cross a boulder field at 1 mile. Notice the hard work volunteers have done to smooth your passage over this rugged section.

Rock formations mark your arrival at Angels Rest at 1.5 miles. Take the short blue-blazed side trail to the right and walk onto the large rock for excellent views of the New River winding through the valley it has created for itself through thousands of years of erosive action. Peters Mountain rises from the far side of the river.

Return to the A.T., continue to ascend, and pass a side trail to a spring and campsite at 2 miles. The rock ledge to the left at 2.1 miles overlooks the New River, wide Wilburn Valley dotted by farmlands and small settlements, and Sugar Run and Salt Pond Mountains to the east.

The walking is quite easy for the next several miles as the A.T. stays along the broad crest of Pearis Mountain. Trillium and mayapple are abundant in early spring. Pass under a power line at 4.1 miles, descend for just a short distance and continue with gradual ups and downs. Doc's Knob Shelter is 100 feet to the west of the Trail at 7.3 miles, while a blue-blazed trail at 8.1 miles leads 150 feet to a view of Sugar Run Mountain.

Cross three dirt roads within the next 3 miles, and swing left on the A.T. at the intersection with the Ribble Trail at 11.2 miles. Watch for the white blazes to direct you through a couple of turns on old woods roads lined by bloodroot, trillium, mayapple, spring beauty, and bluets in springtime. A rock outcrop at 13.4 miles looks north onto Pearis Mountain, which serves as the backdrop for the green fields of the Wilburn Valley.

Begin to descend about a mile from the overlook, cross a branch of Dismal Creek at 15.2 miles, and pass the short side trail to Wapiti Shelter at 15.8 miles. As you walk along, try to imagine yourself transported back a few hundred years to learn of the origin of the shelter's name. At that time, you could have caught sight of a herd of wapiti—the Native American word for elk—grazing in the forest around you. Although they were extirpated from Virginia more than a century ago, a few elk would have been seen here in the 1950s during a failed attempt to reestablish them in the area.

Soon, pass by a small pond, and then the southern intersection with the Ribble Trail at 17.6 miles. Be alert at 20.9 miles as the A.T. makes a sudden left away from the creek. Be alert again in just 0.6 mile, as you want to turn right onto the blue-blazed side trail that leads 0.2 mile to Dismal Creek Falls. The waterfall is not only pretty to look at, but the swimming is great in the creek at its base.

Return to the A.T., skirt the southern slope of Brush Mountain, and come to Virginia 606 at 23.8 miles.

TRAILHEAD DIRECTIONS

To reach the southern trailhead, drive 12 miles east of Bland, Virginia, on Virginia 41 to the intersection with VA 606. Turn left and follow VA 606 0.75 mile to the trailhead.

From Business US 460/Virginia 100 in Pearisburg, turn onto Johnston Avenue. Take the first right onto Morris Avenue and follow it to the northern trailhead in about 1 mile.

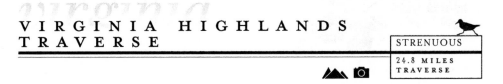

VIRGINIA HIGHLANDS TRAVERSE

STRENUOUS

24.8 MILES
TRAVERSE

Mountain peaks and high meadows are the highlights of this traverse on the "rooftop of Virginia." By taking a side 1-mile round-trip to the fir and spruce-covered summit of Mount Rogers, you will be able to take in Virginia's three highest points on this trip (Rogers, Whitetop, and Pine Mountains). Mount Rogers was known as Balsam Mountain until 1883, when it was named for William Barton Rogers (1804-1882). Rogers was Virginia's first state geologist. Mount Rogers' summit is covered with red spruce and the northernmost stand of fraser fir.

The open fields at Grayson Highlands, Wilburn Ridge, Rhododendron Gap, Pine Mountain, and Buzzard Rocks offer many sweeping panoramas that are without peer in the southeast United States.

This popular area attracts hikers, particularly from mid-June to the first week in July, when the hundreds of acres of rhododendrons along the Trail burst into bloom. The awesome spectacle of the vast fields in bloom is a must-see display. These same meadows are filled with ripe blueberries in late August, but fewer hikers attend that event.

Three miles of this hike pass through Grayson Highlands State Park, where ponies roam free along the Trail. The ponies aren't actually wild, but feral, having been placed here in the early part of the twentieth century. Some of them are sold at auction during a fall festival to raise money to care for the rest of the herd. Although the ponies may approach you, it is best that you neither approach nor attempt to ride them.

This traverse is crossed many times by other trails that form a number of possible loop hikes for both hikers and horseback riders. Be careful and follow the white-blazed A.T. at all times. In the high meadows, the Trail is marked with blazes on fence posts.

Much of this hike is over 4,000 feet in elevation, and the temperature can be cool even in the summer. Be prepared for extremes in weather, particularly as you hike or camp in open areas.

THE HIKE

From the trailhead on Virginia 603, hike south, enter the woods, and begin climbing along the northern slope of Pine Mountain. In 0.2 mile, you will enter the Lewis Fork Wilderness Area. At mile 0.9, cross the Old Orchard Horse Trail, and at mile 1.6, cross the Lewis Fork Horse Trail. In another 0.1 mile, reach Old Orchard Shelter. Water is available from a nearby spring.

Beyond the shelter, the Trail continues to climb Pine Mountain. In 0.5 mile, leave the wilderness area. At mile 3.4, reach the highpoint on the open crest of Pine Mountain (elevation 4,900 feet), where a blue-blazed trail leads off to the right. Enjoy the magnificent views here.

Descend gradually from Pine Mountain to a rail-fenced corral known as "The Scales" at mile 4.8. The name comes from this spot's historical use as a weighing and loading station for cattle. Pass through the fences and begin climbing the northwest slope of Stone Mountain. In 0.3 mile, reach the open summit of Stone Mountain (elevation 4,800 feet).

Descend 0.9 mile to the entrance to the Little Wilson Creek Wilderness Area, which the Trail passes through for the next 1.2 miles. At mile 7.3, cross the East Fork of Big Wilson Creek. At mile 7.5, cross Little Wilson Creek, as you enter Grayson Highlands State Park. Camping and campfires are not permitted, but you are permitted to spend the night in Wise Shelter, which you will pass at 7.6 miles. In another 0.9 mile, cross a stile over a fence and then cross Quebec Branch. In 1.3 miles, reach the junction with the blue-blazed Rhododendron Trail. Hike 0.5 mile beyond this trail junction to the rail fence marking the boundary of Grayson Highlands State Park. Cross a stile and enter Jefferson National Forest. In 0.3 mile, reach the junction with the Wilburn Ridge Trail.

Continue following the A.T., and at mile 11.9, reach Rhododendron Gap (elevation 5,440 feet) at the heart of hundreds of acres of rhododendrons. Two blue-blazed trails intersect the A.T. in the Gap. Follow the white blazes across the mountain, and reenter the Lewis Fork Wilderness Area. The A.T. passes through the wilderness area for the next 3.5 miles.

At mile 12.7, reach Thomas Knob Shelter. Water is available from a nearby spring. Beyond the shelter, hike 0.1 mile to the junction with a blue-blazed side trail. Turn right and follow this pathway for 0.5 mile to the summit of Mount Rogers (elevation 5,729 feet), Virginia's highest peak. The mountain supports the northernmost natural stand of Fraser Fir, and boasts an annual rainfall average of 60 inches and snowfall average of 57 inches. Although there is no vista from the summit, the fir-covered peak makes a wonderful picnic spot.

Return to the A.T., and skirt the southeast flank of Mount Rogers. In 1 mile, cross a fence on a stile, and in another 0.7 mile, reach the junctions with the blue-blazed Mount Rogers Trail and the Virginia Highlands Horse Trail. At mile 15.9, reach the former site of Deep Gap Shelter, which is still on many maps. The shelter is now on display in a park in Damascus, Virginia. In 1.4 miles, cross a fence that marks the wilderness area boundary, and in 0.6 mile, cross Virginia 600, where there is a small parking area. There is also a junction with the Virginia Highlands Horse Trail. Climb along the east slope of Whitetop Mountain.

At mile 20.4, reach the gravel Whitetop Mountain Road, and follow the road briefly. If you would like to make a side trip to the summit of Whitetop (elevation 5,520 feet), continue on the gravel road when the A.T. turns left off of it. It is about 0.25 mile to the top.

Leave Whitetop Mountain Road, pass by an excellent spring, and cross a high meadow on the way to Buzzard Rocks at mile 21.1, which offer a commanding view of the valley below. Descend steeply from Buzzard Rocks, often over switchbacks, and cross Virginia 601 at mile 23.6. Continue, with a few small uphill sections, on this mostly downhill hike and reach the end of the trip, US 58, at mile 24.8.

Trailhead Directions

The northern trailhead is a parking area on VA 603 about 4 miles west of Troutdale, Virginia. The southern trailhead is on US 58, 0.4 mile east of Summit Cut, and 14 miles east of Damascus, Virginia.

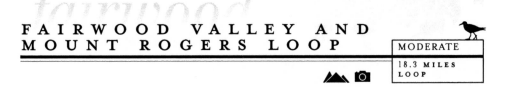

FAIRWOOD VALLEY AND MOUNT ROGERS LOOP

MODERATE

18.3 MILES
LOOP

This loop hike covers some of the most varied terrain in the Southern Appalachians—fields and forests, open meadows covered with rhododendrons and blueberries, and spruce and fir atop Mount Rogers. Mount Rogers, whose summit is visited via a side trail, is the highest point in Virginia (elevation 5,729 feet). Snow can still be seen atop the summit as late as March. In addition to Mount Rogers, this hike features Pine Mountain (elevation 5,050 feet), a high plateau of open meadows dotted with trees, rock outcroppings, rhododendrons, and azaleas.

THE HIKE

The outing commences by crossing VA 603, walking into the woods on the blue-blazed Mount Rogers Trail and taking the boardwalk over a wet area crowded with great rhododendrons. Immediately begin the climb that will last for several miles.

The Trail to the right at 0.4 mile leads to the forest service's Grindstone Campground; stay to the left and use a series of short footbridges to step over small water runs. At 0.9 mile, negotiate the first of a number of switchbacks as your climb runs along a pathway bordered by ferns, gnarled beech trees, Indian pipe, and star moss. Forming compact mats, mosses are capable of storing large amounts of moisture, making them an important part of the forest during times of drought. Coming onto a natural shelf amidst

a younger forest, the ascent levels out for a bit; bypass the Lewis Fork Spur Trail, which comes in from the left at 2.4 miles.

Conspicuous crimson bee balm flowers grow in a wet area at 3.6 miles during the summer, while Turk's cap lily rises beside the Trail around 3.8 miles. Unless the route has been recently maintained, expect to have legs scratched where nettles and thorn bushes droop over the treadway around 4.1 miles. The water you hear, but can't see, is an underground system close to the surface.

The Mount Rogers Trail comes to an end at 4.25 miles; turn left and continue ascending, now along the white-blazed Appalachian Trail. The first of the vistas come into view as you break out of the vegetation to look upon Whitetop Mountain to the southwest. Be sure to swing to the left at 5.25 miles and not go through the stile into the meadow on your right. Walk into open fields again at 5.9 miles, now understanding why you huffed and puffed for so long. With almost no signs of modern civilization, alpine meadows gradually slope away from you, furnishing dazzling views across Helton Creek Valley and onto some of North Carolina's highest mountains.

When the Mount Rogers National Recreation Area was established in 1966, some people saw it as a way to develop the region and proposed that a major ski resort, complete with multiple runs, lifts, and condominiums be constructed in the high country. Thankfully, for those of us who like our recreation areas more natural, those ideas faded away.

Bear left onto the blue-blazed trail at 6.2 miles and make the final push to the state's highest point. The rich perfume of fir and spruce are an olfactory delight when the pathway enters the forest at 6.5 miles. White wood sorrel blossoms, with their shamrock-shaped leaves, dot the thick mats of green moss, which cover the trailside boulders.

Negotiate several rock steps and, at 6.7 miles, arrive on the summit, marked by a USGS triangulation plaque on the highest rock within the state of Virginia. There may be no view from here, but the rustling sound of the wind, the flow of a variety of bird songs, the continuous hum of dozens of insects, and the wonderful aroma of the forest will entice you to tarry.

In 1840, William Barton Rogers, head of the University of Virginia's natural philosophy department, was hired by the commonwealth as the state's first geologist and commissioned to explore the highlands region. Walking onto what he called "Balsam Mountain," Rogers sent back glowing reports about the area's resources. Soon after his death in 1882, the Virginia legislature honored him by declaring the summit would bear his name.

Return to the A.T. and turn left, coming to Thomas Knob Shelter at 7.6 miles. Check out the boulders behind it, where you can enjoy a repeat performance of the vistas you surveyed earlier in the day. Continue your journey along the A.T., reaching the top of a knob in 0.5 mile, where a whole new world opens up. Say goodbye to the Mount Rogers ridgeline and gaze out upon the expanse of Wilburn Ridge and Grayson Highlands State Park.

Pass through a fence and come into a semi-open area at 8.3 miles. The Pine Mountain Trail comes in from the left at 8.6 miles. Keep to the right on the A.T., but less than 100 feet later, bear left onto the Crest Trail, breaking out into the open and descending along switchbacks.

Begin to rise at 9 miles and follow Pine Mountain's undulations to a knoll at 9.8 miles. The Lewis Fork Trail comes in from the left, but stay to the right along the Crest Trail, entering a 600-foot long rhododendron thicket at 9.9 miles. Top a short rise at 10.7 miles; be sure to stay on the Crest Trail, even though the white blazes of the A.T. become visible to the left. Buttercups, Queen Anne's lace, and a mint (known as heal all) populate the meadow as you descend and turn left onto the A.T. at 11.7 miles. Toilets and The Scales, once a cattle weighing station, are just below you at this point.

Enter a forest of yellow birch and red spruce at 11.9 miles and pass through a fence. Just a few miles south of here (on Whitetop Mountain), the red spruce reaches its natural southern limit. Swing to the left at 12.6 miles, begin the climb back to the Pine Mountain crest, pass through another fence at 12.9 miles, and come into a semi-open area with high blueberry bushes.

You should take a short side trip to the rocks on your left to view the Mount Rogers ridgeline and much of the terrain you have already traversed. Return and continue along the A.T. Reenter the woods and pass by the blue-blazed Pine Mountain Trail at 13.1 miles; you are now standing at an elevation of exactly 5,000 feet above sea level. Leave the open areas, descend into woods and, at 14.8 miles, reach Old Orchard Shelter, which overlooks the crest of Iron Mountain to the west.

Continue on the A.T for 0.1 mile, bear left onto the Old Orchard Spur Trail, and in 0.3 mile, turn right to descend along the Lewis Fork Trail. Avoiding the Cliffside

Trail to the left at 16.1 miles, keep right and continue along the Lewis Fork Trail, dropping at a barely perceptible rate along the creek. Bee balm covers the banks of Lewis Fork, which you cross on a footbridge. Keep to the left onto a lesser-used route just a few hundred feet later as the horse trail veers right. Be sure to turn around and gaze upon all of the elevation you have lost since leaving the highlands.

Cross VA 603 at 17 miles. There may be no discernible pathway, but continue straight across the field, aiming for the trees in front of you. Copious amounts of clover, Queen Anne's lace, heal all, daisy, aster, and buttercup bring color to the meadow.

Turn left onto the Fairwood Valley Trail at 17.1 miles, pass through a fence and enter the woods. Cross a small water run in 0.1 mile and make the final little uphill incline of the hike. Thousands of roots exposed by the cut of this woods road show what an extensive support network trees have hidden underground.

Begin a gradual descent at 17.8 miles, keep left when a trail rises to the right and, at 18.1 miles, return to the car you walked away from when you began this hike.

TRAILHEAD DIRECTIONS

Drive to the trailhead by taking I-81 Exit 45 in Marion and heading south on VA 16, passing by the Mount Rogers National Recreation Area Visitor Center in 6.1 miles. Continue for another 11.2 miles to Troutdale where you turn right onto VA 603. The trailhead parking is identified by a small sign on the right 5.7 miles later.

BECAUSE SO MANY MILES OF THE A.T. TRAVERSE THE
TENNESSEE–NORTH CAROLINA BORDER, THESE TWO
STATES ARE USUALLY PLACED TOGETHER IN TRAIL
GUIDES. COMBINED, THE TWO STATES OFFER MORE
THAN 370 MILES OF TRAIL. HEADING SOUTH, THE TRAIL
BEGINS IN TENNESSEE (HEADING NORTH, IT BEGINS IN
NORTH CAROLINA).

Tennessee and North Carolina

FOR THE FIRST 37 MILES, THE TRAIL TRAVERSES THE
RIDGELINE AS IT MAKES ITS WAY TO WATAUGA LAKE
NEAR HAMPTON, TENNESSEE. FROM HAMPTON, THE
TRAIL HEADS THROUGH LAUREL FORK GORGE,
WHERE THERE ARE SPECTACULAR WATERFALLS, AND
CONTINUES UP WHITE ROCKS MOUNTAIN BEFORE IT
DESCENDS TO ELK PARK, NORTH CAROLINA.

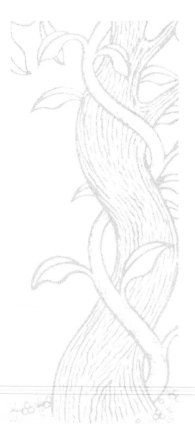

FROM ELK PARK, A STRENUOUS CLIMB PAST THE
HUMP MOUNTAINS LEADS TO GRASSY RIDGE (A
6,000-FOOT GRASSY BALD), ROAN HIGHLANDS, ROAN
HIGH KNOB, AND ROAN HIGH BLUFF. ROAN HIGH
BLUFF, OVER 6,000 FEET HIGH, IS KNOWN FOR ITS
SPECTACULAR RHODODENDRON GARDENS THAT
BLOOM PROFUSELY EACH JUNE. FROM ROAN, THE
TRAIL CONTINUES ALONG THE TENNESSEE–NORTH

Carolina border for nearly 100 miles as it makes its way to Hot Springs, North Carolina, and heads into the Great Smoky Mountains National Park. In this section, the Trail passes Little Rock Knob, Unaka Mountain, and Beauty Spot. It descends to Erwin, Tennessee, and then to Hot Springs.

From Hot Springs, it is just over 30 miles to Davenport Gap, the northern entrance of the A.T. into the Smoky Mountains. In the Smokies, the Trail traverses Mount Cammerer, the Sawteeth, and Charlies Bunion, reaches Newfound Gap, and proceeds to Clingmans Dome, the highest point on the entire A.T. (elevation 6,643 feet).

The A.T. continues across Silers Bald to Thunderhead and Rocky Top, and down to Spence and Russell Fields, continues to Shuckstack, before descending to Fontana Dam at the Little Tennessee River, the southern boundary of the Great Smoky Mountains National Park.

From the Smokies, the A.T. ascends into the Nantahalas with its 4,000 and 5,000-foot peaks. From the Nantahala Outdoor Center at Wesser, the A.T. climbs up to Wesser Bald, Wayah Bald, and Silers Bald, then heads up to the ridge along Standing Indian Mountain. Albert Mountain is also a notable climb in this section. From Albert, it is not far to the North Carolina/ Georgia border at Bly Gap.

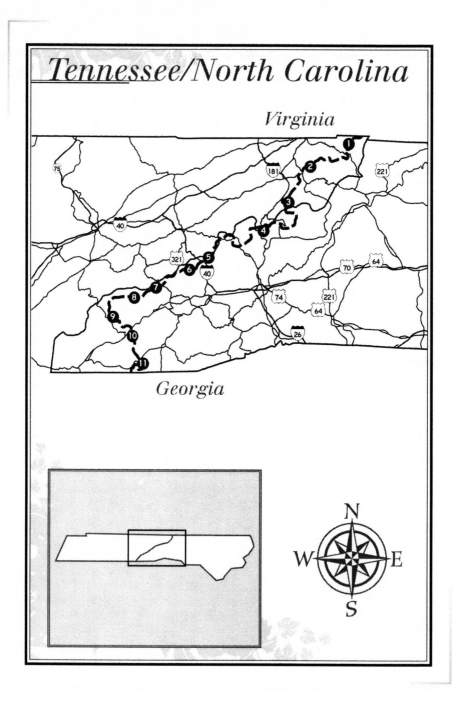

Tennessee/North Carolina

Virginia

Georgia

IRON MOUNTAIN
TRAVERSE

EASY

19.9 MILES
TRAVERSE

This traverse follows the narrow ridge-line of Iron Mountain, passing through nearly 6 miles of the Big Laurel Branch Wilderness Area. The Trail offers many fine views of Watauga Lake, which is located just below the steep southern slope of Iron mountain.

On this hike, you will also pass a monument to Nick Grindstaff (1851-1923). He was a local hermit who, as noted on his monument, "lived alone, suffered alone, died alone." The marker is made from the remains of the chimney to his cabin.

The last part of this hike can often be overgrown by midsummer. The volunteer trail maintainers have difficulty keeping up with the quick-growing weeds. Iron Mountain is particularly nice when the leaves have fallen in preparation for winter because it offers many more views. Although rated as easy, remember that no 20-mile hike on the A.T. is without significant climbs and descents.

THE HIKE

From the Trailhead on Tennessee 91, hike south and begin a moderate ascent. Cross a logging road at mile 0.4. The Trail in this section crosses a couple of wet areas on bog bridges. Continue to ascend Iron Mountain steadily, reaching a highpoint at mile 2.7.

At mile 3.2, locate the Nick Grindstaff Monument. It is the stone chimney a short distance to your right. The inscription does not face the Trail. In another 1.3 miles, reach Iron Mountain Shelter. Water is available from a small stream about 0.25 mile beyond the shelter. Reach another highpoint on the ridge about 0.5 mile beyond the shelter.

At mile 5.3, cross under power lines in a utility right-of-way, and enjoy year-round views. In 0.4 mile, cross over another highpoint on the ridge, and in another 0.25 mile, reach the junction with an unnamed blue-blazed trail. Continue following the A.T. and reach Turkeypen Gap at mile 6.2. For the next mile, there are several unblazed trails leading off the ridge. Continue following the white blazes across the ridge top. At mile 8.2, reach the junction with the Horselog Ridge Trail, and at mile 9.9, enter the Big Laurel Branch Wilderness Area. The remainder of the hike is in this wilderness area.

Reach Vandeventer Shelter at mile 11.2. Water is available from a spring located down a blue-blazed trail, which branches off the A.T. a short distance beyond the shelter. The blue-blazed trail leads 0.5 mile down the mountain to a spring, so it is a good idea to bring water with you to the shelter, if possible. Behind the shelter, a rock outcrop offers a particularly good view of Watauga Lake.

About 1.5 miles past the shelter, the Trail begins its descent from Iron Mountain. It is a steady descent from here to the lake. At mile 16, reach Watauga Dam Road.

Climb the stone steps, reenter the woods, and ascend to a highpoint at mile

16.6. Then descend sharply for 0.25 mile to join the access road that leads to the dam. Follow the road as it descends to and crosses Watauga Lake Dam. At mile 18.2, reach the short blue-blazed side trail to Watauga Lake Shelter. Water is available from the creek that the Trail crosses on the way to the shelter.

At mile 19.1, cross a dirt road, which to the left leads to a beach on the lake. In another 0.3 mile, pass around a steel gate. The Trail then passes between the lake to the left and houses to the right. At mile 19.9, reach the USFS Shook Branch Recreation Area, the end of this hike.

TRAILHEAD DIRECTIONS

Locate the northern trailhead on TN 91, 19 miles north of Elizabethton, Tennessee, and 4 miles south of US 421 in Shady Valley, Tennessee. Locate the southern trailhead at the USFS Shook Branch Recreation Area on US 321, about 3 miles east of Hampton, Tennessee.

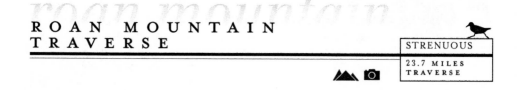

ROAN MOUNTAIN TRAVERSE

STRENUOUS

23.7 MILES TRAVERSE

This hike features a walk along the crest of the Iron Mountains. The A.T. winds its way over knolls and balds from Indian Grave Gap to the spectacular summit of Roan Mountain. Unaka Bald (elevation 5,180 feet) and Little Rock Knob (elevation 4,919 feet) are also notable features on this overnight hike.

If this hike is taken in mid to late June, the highlight will be the Cloudland rhododendron gardens atop Roan Mountain. Every year, the beautiful Catawba rhododendrons burst into bloom, carpeting the mountain with their purple flowers. Don't be surprised, though, to find the mountain socked in with fog. The elevation of Roan—6,285 feet at Roan High Knob—means the summit is often capped by clouds. Fraser fir and red spruce also abound atop Roan.

The hike ends at Carvers Gap, opposite Grassy Ridge, the only 6,000-plus-foot bald on the A.T.

THE HIKE

From Indian Grave Gap (elevation 3,360 feet), enter the woods on the north side of the road. In 0.75 mile, you will reach a cut-through and join an abandoned road. As you continue, other abandoned roads will cross the Trail.

Nearly 0.5 mile later, cross the gravel USFS 230 and begin to climb along the right side of the ridge. Reach the crest of the ridge in 0.1 mile, turn left, and continue to climb. At about mile 2, enter an open field, continue along a road track, and turn right. You will soon head left around a knoll and follow the A.T. through a sag.

Almost 0.5 mile later, you will reach the summit of Beauty Spot (elevation 4,437 feet), at mile 2.3 of the hike. This grassy bald has great views of Roan Mountain to the east, the Black Mountains to the south, Big Bald and the Flattop Mountains to the southwest, and the Toe River Valley below. You might also catch several glimpses of the Nolichucky River to the south and west.

The A.T. continues along an old road track then leaves the field and road, entering the woods. In 0.25 mile, you will reach Beauty Spot Gap (elevation 4,300 feet) at a gate in a fence where USFS 230 enters from the left. The blue-blazed trail leads a short distance through the gate and across the road to a spring. There is a good campsite on a small knoll to the east. Continue to the right on the A.T., keeping to the left of the fence. A short distance from the end of the fence, head straight downhill a short ways, then head left and continue to descend.

Hike 0.1 mile to where the Trail levels out and turns left, then cross a small bog in 0.25 mile. A side trail, just before the bog, leads a short distance to a spring and campsite, and further to USFS 230. Climb along the ridge, cross an old woods road, and enter the woods again. In 0.5 mile, you will see a field to your right and a road to your left. Head away from the road and soon cross a small summit.

Reach Deep Gap (elevation 4,100 feet) at mile 3.8. There is a good campsite in the meadow to your left. Just across the road, an old, graded trail leads to a spring boxed with concrete. A trail at the western end of the gap heads right 1.2 miles to Upper Poplar. When the road heads left to skirt left of the summit of Unaka Mountain, leave the road and begin to climb the ridge toward the summit of Unaka.

In 0.5 mile, at a switchback on the crest, USFS 230 is only a few feet to the left. Continue up the Trail along switchbacks. In another 0.25 mile, you will reach the crest and continue to climb gradually through the woods, crossing a quartzite ledge as you reach the broad summit area.

Reach the benchmark on the summit of Unaka Mountain (elevation 5,180 feet) at mile 5.4. From this evergreen woods with its rare stand of red spruce, descend to hardwoods, then steeply off the mountain. You will pass a spring and continue your steep descent. Hike 1.5 miles to a trail junction. The Trail is unmarked but leads about 0.5 mile to USFS 230; it is also the former route of the A.T. Turn sharply to the right on the A.T., and skirt the to the left of the ridge.

At Low Gap (elevation 3,900 feet), just over 0.25 mile later, a poorly defined side trail leads a short distance to a spring just to the right of the Trail at the base of a hemlock tree. The A.T. follows the Tennessee–North Carolina border for the next 4 miles. The Trail continues from Low Gap, climbing to the east.

Reach Cherry Gap Shelter at mile 8.1. Water is available from a good piped spring on a blue-blazed trail. From the shelter, continue along the ridge crest for nearly 0.5 mile to Cherry Gap (elevation 3,900 feet). A woods road passes through the gap heading left to USFS 230 and right to Pigeonroost, North Carolina. The Trail climbs out of the gap, and in 0.25 mile, skirts the southern slope of Piney Bald. The open summit affords good views. To reach the summit, you must bushwhack through the woods.

Continue along the A.T., head right into a narrow gap within 0.25 mile, and climb steeply up the ridge. In just over 0.25 mile, cross the left shoulder of a small knob, turn left, and descend through the woods. The A.T. then mostly follows the ridge crest with gentle ups and downs. At mile 9.6, you will reach the summit of Little Bald Knob (elevation 4,459 feet).

From the summit, descend the ridge with a fence to your left. At the edge of the woods, you should be able to see Roan

Mountain. In 0.25 mile, cross an old logging road, pass to the left of a big rock outcropping, descend steeply, and cross a graded trail. Hike 0.1 mile to a sag where underbrush may slightly obscure the Trail. Begin to climb again, closing in on the fence to your right. You will then head right, away from the ridge crest, and descend along the footpath.

Reach an old woods road in 0.25 mile, and turn left onto a gravel road in another 0.25 mile. The A.T. follows the gravel road for a short distance and returns to the woods, heading along the right side of the ridgeline. The gravel road parallels the Trail, above, on the crest. At mile 10.8, reach Iron Mountain Gap (elevation 3,723 feet) at Tennessee 107/ North Carolina 226. A grocery store with limited supplies for hikers is 0.5 mile to your right.

From here, the A.T. passes through a gate and climbs along a gravel road, along the left side of the ridge crest, for the next 1.5 miles. In nearly 0.5 mile, a fence and tree farm border the road to the left. There are good views here back toward Unaka Mountain. In another 0.5 mile, the woods on your right end just below the summit, and afford spectacular views of Unaka to the west, Roan to the southeast, and Little Rock Knob to the east. Leave the crest and head downhill along the road.

Soon, an old track will come in from the right; keep to the left and continue to descend along the road. At mile 12, enter an old orchard, continuing along the road, and pass through a slight saddle, skirting the right side of a knoll. Take care to note when the A.T. turns off the road. While the road continues ahead, descending the Tennessee side of the mountain, the A.T. heads east through the woods, turning right and descending into a weedy gap.

After the gap, enter the woods, begin to climb again, and shortly thereafter, turn left uphill. A blue-blazed side trail descends steeply to the right for 0.1 mile to a stream. In 0.25 mile, reach the crest of the ridge, which the Trail follows for the next 2 miles. Continue to climb beside a fence and enjoy occasional views to your left. In just under 0.5 mile, top the first major summit of the ridge, and 0.25 mile later, reach the second summit (elevation 4,426 feet). From here, continue along the ridge top and soon pass an overhanging rock.

Hike another 1.25 mile to the summit of a knob (elevation 4,332 feet), and then head left. Descend along the inside edge of the woods with a wire fence and field to your right. From the field, view Roan High Bluff and Grassy Ridge to the south and southeast. In just over 0.25 mile, reach the corner of the old field and begin to descend gradually along the ridge crest. At mile 14.6, reach a blue-blazed side trail that descends steeply to a spring and campsite. The side trail continues past the campsite and joins the A.T. again at Greasy Creek Gap.

The A.T. reaches Greasy Creek Gap (elevation 4,034 feet) in another 0.25 mile. To the right, a dirt road descends to Buladean, North Carolina, and to the left, 2.5 miles to Tiger Creek. From the gap, the A.T. continues straight ahead along an old woods road, climbing the ridge crest for the next 1.8 miles. Nearly a mile from the gap, reach the foundation of old homestead with a row of six maple trees in front. There is a spring a short distance down the hollow to the left. Continue between the homestead and the row of trees.

At mile 16.5, reach a shallow gap; the Trail runs parallel to an old road on the right. In 0.25 mile, a road to the left leads a short distance to a spring. The A.T. heads away from the road and becomes a treadway. In another 0.1 mile, you will reach the blue-blazed side trail that heads left a short distance to the Clyde Smith Shelter. Water is available from a spring a short distance behind the shelter. The sign for the shelter is hard to see, and the shelter is not visible from the Trail.

From the side trail for the shelter, the A.T. continues to climb through trees and a grassy area, eventually skirting the left side of a knoll near the edge of the woods, just below the summit. The partly open summit (elevation 4,640 feet) can be reached by hiking a short distance to your right. Begin to descend along the ridge crest, reaching a gap in another 0.25 mile. A side trail in the gap heads left for 0.1 mile to a spring. From the gap, begin to climb again through a hardwood forest.

In just over 0.25 mile, you will enter a rhododendron and laurel grove and continue to climb steeply along a narrow path as you ascend toward Little Rock Knob. Reach the cliffs of the knob in 0.1 mile. Little Rock Knob (elevation 4,918 feet) offers spectacular views to the west and north. The A.T. continues through rhododendron and laurel just below the summit before heading right and descending steeply off the southern slope.

Enter a field in a gap with young tree growth 0.75 mile later. Climb steeply with a new fence to your left. On the other side of the fence is a wooded area with lots of blowdowns (chestnuts). In another 0.25 mile, pass over a summit, and beyond a slight gap, the Trail widens into an old woods road. Pass over a second summit in another 0.25 mile, and reach the road crossing at Hughes Gap (elevation 4,040 feet) at mile 18.9. The A.T. continues across the road to the left.

On the north side of the road, the A.T. climbs steeply up the left side of the ridge along an old road. Hike 0.5 mile to where the Trail returns to the ridge crest and begin to climb to Cloudland. At mile 20.2, reach a side trail that heads right to an overlook with good views. From the side trail, hike 0.1 mile to the summit of Beartown Mountain (elevation 5,481 feet), and then descend through a beech wood. Hike nearly 0.5 mile further to Ash Gap

(elevation 5,340 feet) where there is a good campsite. A very faint trail leads 0.1 mile to a small spring.

Continue along the A.T. for just over 0.5 mile to an area of dense spruce and rhododendrons. Turn left off the old trail 0.1 mile later, begin to climb steeply, and reach a summit (elevation 6,150 feet) in another 0.1 mile. Turn right and enter a grassy meadow that leads to an open area. Look straight ahead to locate the former site of the Cloudland Hotel. There are excellent views of the Black Mountains from here. Next to the former hotel site is a small forest service parking lot, and to the right, a larger forest service parking lot. Beyond these parking lots are the Cloudland rhododendron gardens and drinking water from fountains. To the west, view Roan High Bluff (elevation 6,267 feet).

From here, descend a rocky bank to the left of the path to the parking lot, and follow an old road track to the large spruce tree at the left front comer of the hotel site. At mile 21.6, you will turn left and enter the woods. Not long thereafter, you will reach an old cabin site. Head right, cross toward the opposite corner, head left beyond the site, and descend through the woods.

In 0.1 mile, pass a picnic table at the edge of a road. Keep left and follow the old road (don't cross the paved road) through Fraser fir and rhododendrons. The A.T. follows this road nearly all the way to Carvers Gap.

In 0.5 mile, reach a blue-blazed trail to your right that leads 0.1 mile to the summit of Roan High Knob (elevation 6,285 feet), at mile 22.2 of the hike. The summit of Roan High Knob boasts the highest shelter on the A.T. Formerly a fire warden's cabin, the shelter was renovated in 1980 for hiker use. Water is available from a spring behind the cabin on a blue-blazed trail.

The A.T. continues along the old road, skirting the left side of a knob. Beyond the knob, descend along several switchbacks.

Just over a mile later, turn left off the road onto a footpath and descend. Head to the right through weeds and a stand of open fir. In 0.1 mile, you will reach the paved USFS Cloudland Rhododendron Garden Road near a large rock. The Trail heads left downhill to the left of a pole fence.

At mile 23.7, reach Carvers Gap (elevation 5,512 feet), the end of this hike. To your left, locate a parking lot and a picnic area with spring and toilets.

TRAILHEAD DIRECTIONS

From Erwin, Tennessee, reach Indian Grave Gap via Tennessee 395 (10th Street in Erwin; Rock Creek Road outside the city limits). The A.T. crossing is 6.6 miles southeast of Erwin. At mile 3.3, you will reach the USFS Rock Creek Recreation Area.

Reach Carvers Gap via Tennessee 143, 14 miles south of Roan Mountain, Tennessee, or via North Carolina 261, 14 miles north of Bakersville, North Carolina.

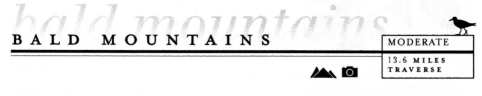

BALD MOUNTAINS

MODERATE

13.6 MILES
TRAVERSE

The summits of High Rocks and Big Bald are the highlights of this short traverse over the Bald Mountains. High Rocks is on a short side trail off the A.T. and affords great views of Little Bald, Temple Hill, and No Business Knob. Big Bald offers spectacular 360 degree views of the Southern Appalachians, including an excellent view of Mount Mitchell only 20 miles distant. Mitchell (elevation 6,684 feet) is the highest peak east of Mississippi River and lies in the Black Mountains of North Carolina. Mount LeConte in the Great Smoky Mountains can also be seen from Big Bald. To the southwest, between the Black Mountains and the Smoky Mountains, view the Nantahala Mountains; to the northwest, view Coldspring Mountain with its two peaks, Camp Creek Bald and Big Butt; and to the northeast, view the Unaka Mountains.

After ascending from Sams Gap, the A.T. crosses extensive open pastures and follows the ridge crest to Street Gap where the A.T. begins a long, gradual climb up Big Bald (elevation 5,516 feet). From the extensive meadows at Big Bald, the A.T. descends to the Bald Mountain Shelter, makes the short climb up the wooded summit of Little Bald, descends to Whistling Gap, and then climbs to High Rocks. The traverse ends at Spivey Gap, just north of US 19W.

THE HIKE

From Sams Gap (elevation 3,800 feet), follow the white-blazed A.T. south. At mile 1, in a slight sag, find an intermittent spring to your left. A short distance later, you will pass a dirt road that heads left to US 23 in Tennessee. In another 0.1 mile, pass an abandoned talc mine to your right, and continue to climb to the right of a barbed wire fence. Reach the top of a knob (elevation 4,440 feet) at mile 2 of the hike, and leave the woods for open meadows. View Big Bald to the northeast. The Trail continues across the meadow, descending to the left of the fence.

In another 0.25 mile, the fence (and the Trail) heads right. You will skirt a small knob to the left and return to following the fence. At mile 2.6, reach the road at Street Gap (left to Flag Pond; right to a paved road and the first house on Puncheon Fork Road). On the other side of the road, follow a dirt road through the fence and begin to climb along the ridge crest. View Big Bald to your left.

Hike 0.5 mile to where the Trail heads right and the dirt road continues straight up the ridge. Follow this graded trail, switchback to your left, and reach the ridge crest in 0.25 mile. Turn right and descend steeply into the Cherokee National Forest.

At mile 3.7, the A.T. leaves the road and ridgeline, heading left along the Tennessee side of the ridge. In 0.1 mile, reach a blue-blazed trail that heads left a short distance to a spring. Reach Low Gap at mile 4 of the hike.

From Low Gap, climb through hardwoods and a spring wildflower garden for about a mile, passing a spring in just over 0.5 mile. One mile from Low Gap, pass ruins to the left of the Trail, skirt the left slope of the ridge, and climb moderately. Climb gently for a mile and reach a blue-blazed side trail that heads left a short distance to a spring. In another 0.1 mile, reach a blue-blazed trail that leads a very short distance to a spring. The side trail can also be used in bad weather because it follows the southeastern slope of Big Bald on graded trail, turns left on Wolf Laurel Road, and rejoins the A.T. at mile 7 at Big Stamp. Big Bald can be nearly impossible to navigate in foggy or stormy weather.

In another 0.25 mile, begin to climb steeply up a rocky slope, crossing several small streams. A short distance later, enter a rhododendron grove as you continue to climb, and reach more level trail in another 0.25 mile. The Trail bears right and continues up the east slope of Big Bald, soon passing through scattered mountain ash, serviceberry, and hawthorn before entering the open, grassy meadows of the bald.

At mile 6.8, reach the highest point on Big Bald (elevation 5,516 feet), which is marked by a post. From the summit, descend the treeless saddle of Big Stamp. In 0.2 mile, reach the junction with the "bad weather" trail at mile 7. Reach a campsite with double springs in just over 0.25 mile by following the road to the left and taking the right fork. The left fork leads to a grassed over parking lot near the summit.

From this trail junction, climb along the ridge crest and across meadows with great views. Nearly 0.5 mile later, pass over a small rise with scattered trees and large rocks. To the southwest, enjoy an excellent close-up view of Big Bald. In 0.25 mile, descend through an open meadow with a view of Little Bald ahead. Enter the woods, and soon thereafter, cross a dirt road and re-enter the woods.

At mile 7.9, reach a blue-blazed side trail on your left that leads 0.1 mile to Bald Mountain Shelter. At 5,100 ft., this is one of the highest shelter on the A.T. Water is available from a spring down another short side trail between the Trail and the shelter. Camping is not encouraged here because the area around the shelter is very fragile. If you're interested in camping, a good spot is located at mile 8.3.

Cross a small stream in 0.25 mile, and a short distance later, a spring to your right. In another 0.25 mile, reach the junction with another blue-blazed trail that heads left to Big Bald Creek. There are good campsites along the ridge and a good spring less than 0.25 mile down the Trail near the head of Tumbling Creek. The A.T. continues ahead, alternately following an old woods road and a footpath through the woods.

Reach the end of the road in 0.75 mile. The Trail begins to climb up the ridge to the left of a fence. At mile 9.3, reach the wooded summit of Little Bald (elevation 5,185 feet). The A.T. leaves the Tennessee–North Carolina state line and descends into North Carolina for the last 4.3 miles of this hike. A vista opens to the left a short distance from the summit of Little Bald with views of No Business Knob and Temple Hill to the north. The A.T. continues steeply down the mountain with several switchbacks and steps.

In another 0.75 mile, pass a spring to your left, and 0.25 mile later, the former route of the A.T. enters from the right, leading to the summit of Little Bald. A southerly switchback was completed recently here. Watch the blazes. Continue to descend down the ridge with a barbed wire fence to your right. In 0.5 mile, after climbing a slight rise, pass a huge boulder to your left blazed with the A.T. symbol.

At mile 11.2, reach Whistling Gap (elevation 3,840 feet). The far end of the gap can be used as a campsite. A trail to the left leads 0.1 mile to a spring. Beyond it, the old A.T. heads to US 19W, just west of Spivey Gap. The A.T. continues ahead, climb the crest and soon cross a small knob. Reach a sag in just over 0.25 mile, and begin to climb toward High Rocks.

Near the summit of High Rocks, reach the junction of a blue-blazed trail that heads steeply right to the peak of High Rocks (elevation 4,280 feet). This blue-blazed trail goes beneath the northern rim of High Rocks, rejoining the A.T. at mile 12.

Continue on the A.T. and head left. Skirting the base of a rocky cliff, climb to a small saddle with the peak of High Rocks to your right. At mile 12, the blue-blazed trail rejoins the A.T., which heads left, steeply descending along steps and switchbacks. At mile 12.8, cross some small creeks, and 0.3 mile later, reach an area used as a campsite. You will descend along stone steps and then continue descending along an old road.

Enter a stand of white pine and hemlock, and pass to the right of a clearing in another 0.25 mile. Soon thereafter, cross Big Creek and climb up the bank to the highway. At mile 13.6, reach Spivey Gap at US 19W, the end of this hike.

Trailhead Directions

The A.T. crossing at Sams Gap is on US 23, 12 miles north of Mars Hill, North Carolina, 31 miles north of Asheville, North Carolina, and 6 miles south of Flag Pond.

Spivey Gap, on US 19W, is 8 miles south of Erwin, Tennessee, and 43 miles north of Asheville, North Carolina.

STATE LINE TRAVERSE

EASY

20.2 MILES
TRAVERSE

The A.T. shares a treadway with the forest service State Line Trail from Devil Fork Gap to Allen Gap. This circuitous traverse follows mostly ridge crest from Green Ridge to Camp Creek Bald. The crest is partially cleared in many places and offers especially good views from Ballground and Blackstack Cliffs. Bearwallow Gap features a dense rhododendron thicket.

Also of note on this hike is the grave of William and David Shelton atop Coldspring Mountain. David Shelton, and his nephew, William, left their mountain farms in Shelton Laurel, North Carolina, to join the Union cause. While returning for a rendezvous with their families in a cabin atop Coldspring Mountain, the two men and a boy lookout were ambushed by Confederates and killed. They were buried in a single grave atop the mountain. In 1915, two preachers petitioned the federal government for grave markers. They hauled them up the mountain on an ox sled and erected one at each end of the grave. Because the boy lookout was not a soldier, the government did not supply a tombstone for the youth.

THE HIKE

From North Carolina 212 at Devil Fork Gap (elevation 3,107 feet), head south, climbing up steps and turning right into a field. Climb, with a switchback to the right, and reach the ridge. In 0.1 mile, you will turn right and shortly thereafter pass through a fence. The Trail continues ahead through a slight sag and across a ridge, and then descends steps to an old railroad grade.

After following the railroad bed for a short distance, reach a view of Camp Creek Bald (west) and a sweeping panorama of the Bald Mountains to Green Ridge Knob (north). Continue along the railroad bed, descend for just over 0.5 mile, and climb again.

At mile 1.4, reach the ridge and the former route of the A.T., which heads right to Devil Fork Gap. The A.T. continues along the ridge crest, reaching the site of the old Locust Ridge Shelter (removed in 1982) in nearly 0.5 mile. Water is available in a ravine to the left. The A.T. continues beyond the next rise and then skirts the western side of Flint Mountain. Nearly a mile later, you will pass a spring and two streams and then the Flint Mountain Shelter.

Continue along the A.T., cross a ridge in another 0.5 mile, and descend along a narrow path that widens into an old logging road. At mile 3.5, reach Flint Gap (elevation 3,425 feet) and begin to ascend along a graded trail. Nearly 0.5 mile later, turn right onto a dirt road, and shortly thereafter, turn left as you begin to climb the ridge. The Trail follows the road for about 3 miles, climbing steeply up the ridge crest for a short distance before turning off the crest to the left.

Return to the crest of the ridge at mile 4.5, where the old road comes in from the right. Turn left and climb steeply up the slope of Cold Spring Mountain. In 0.25 mile, at the top of the rise, view Green Ridge Knob to your left as you cross the crest of the ridge on Cold Spring Mountain, and then descend into the woods, following an old road and passing through a stand of white pines.

Pass the graves of David and William Shelton and their 15-year-old relative in 0.5 mile. The markers read, "Wm. Shelton, Co. E, 2 N.C. Inf." and "David Shelton, Co. C, 3 N.C. Mtd. Inf." Continue along the crest, passing alternately through overgrown fields and woods, and in 0.25 mile, reach a blue-blazed dirt road that leads downhill to a spring. The road curves left 0.1 mile later, and there is another spring to the right in a ravine. Pass to the left of the summit of Gravel Knob, and skirt another low summit on your right.

At mile 6.7, the Trail abruptly turns southwest, and shortly thereafter leaves the road and enters the woods. On the other side of the road, the blue-blazed Squibb Creek Trail heads east to Ball Ground on the ridge of Rich Mountain and then to Horse Creek Campground in 4.5 miles. Continue along the A.T. for a short distance, and pass a side trail to your right that leads to the rocky outcropping of Big Rock (elevation 4,838 feet), which offers panoramic views of the valley below. You can also see Camp Creek Bald, Big Bald, and Gravel Knob from here.

The A.T. continues along a rocky footpath, eventually descending on big rock steps. At mile 7, cross a dirt road, and shortly thereafter, reach a small knoll with a cleared view. On the right side of the A.T., locate the small stone memorial to Howard E. Bassett of Connecticut. Bassett, a 1968 thru-hiker, died in late 1987 and his ashes were scattered here on April 27, 1988. Cross the road and pass a large rock to the left of the Trail in 0.25 mile. In another 0.25 mile, cross a cleared field along the left side.

Just over 0.5 mile later, leave the field and enter the woods, turning left and descending into North Carolina along switchbacks. In Chestnut Gap (elevation 4,150 feet), the Trail rejoins the road, and shortly thereafter, reaches Jerry Cabin at mile 8.6. Water is available from a good spring a short distance down a side trail near the shelter.

Continue along the A.T. for 0.25 mile, and reach the junction with the Fork Ridge Trail on your left. It is 2 miles down this trail to Big Creek Road and 2 miles farther to Carmen, North Carolina. The A.T. continues along the dirt road for another 0.75 mile to where the road turns to the right, heading 3 miles to Round Knob Spring and Round Knob Campground Road. The A.T. then continues along graded trail to the right of Big Firescald Knob.

At mile 11.1, pass a spring to the left of the Trail and pass through a rhododendron grove. In another 0.75 mile, you will reach the rhododendron "gardens" at Bearwallow Gap. Here, the forest service Whiteoak Flats Trail heads left 2.5 miles to Hickey Fork Road. The A.T. continues through the rhododendrons for 0.25 mile to the junction with a wide side trail that leads a short distance to Blackstack Cliffs, which offers great views of Tennessee. The A.T. forks left and continues through rhododendrons.

In another 0.25 mile, a side trail heads left a short distance to White Rock Cliffs, a rock outcropping with good views, particularly of the Black Mountains and Mount Mitchell (elevation 6,684 feet). A short descent along switchbacks offers good views to the south and east. Pass a spring to the left of the Trail in 0.1 mile, and continue along the A.T. below the developed Jones Meadow.

Nearly a mile later, reach an old lumber road, which shortly joins with Camp Creek Bald Fire Road. Follow the old lumber road to the left, and within the next 0.1 mile, turn right uphill. There is a spring to the right of the Trail a short distance later. Continue to the left, climbing the eastern ridge of Camp Creek Bald, and circle just below the summit through a thick growth of rhododendrons. Reach another trail junction at mile 14. This trail heads left down Seng Ridge to Pounding Mill Trail, Whiteoak Flats Trail, and Shelton Laurel Road. To the right, the Trail leads 0.25 mile to Camp Creek Bald fire tower (elevation 4,844 feet), which offers great views of the Smokies.

The A.T. continues, descending slightly. Reach Little Laurel Shelter to your left at mile 15.3. Water is available from a boxed spring down the blue-blazed trail to your right. The Trail to the spring is also the start of the Dixon Trail, which heads 1.5 miles to the Camp Creek Bald Fire Road. The A.T. continues to descend, reaching a fork in the Trail in another 2 miles.

Take the left fork (the former route of the A.T. is straight ahead) and in just over 0.25 mile, cross Old Hayesville Road in a stand of white pine. Begin to climb, switchbacking to the left around a hill. In another 0.25 mile, pass a blocked trail to your right, and descend to your left. Hike nearly 0.5 mile to return to the crest in a sag, and cross an old dirt road. Take the right fork of the Trail, climb uphill, and in 0.1 mile, turn left onto the Trail coming up the ridge and continue to climb.

At mile 19.6, turn right, away from the route of the former A.T., continue along the ridge, and reach Allen Gap at Tennessee 70 in 0.6 mile.

TRAILHEAD DIRECTIONS

The A.T. crossing at Devil Fork Gap is on the Tennessee–North Carolina border. From Erwin, Tennessee, reach Devil Fork Gap by taking US 23 south for 12 miles to Rocky Fork and then Tennessee 352 for 4.2 miles to Devil Fork Gap.

To reach the Trail crossing at Allen Gap, take TN 70 for 25 miles south of Greeneville, Tennessee, or by taking US 25W/70 for 6 miles east of Hot Springs, North Carolina, and then North Carolina 208 north 9 miles to Allen Gap.

MAX PATCH AND HOT SPRINGS

MODERATE

19.9 MILES TRAVERSE

This hike offers some tremendous views from the top of Max Patch and takes you over Walnut and Bluff Mountains on the hike into Hot Springs, North Carolina. Max Patch is the southernmost open, grassy bald on the A.T., and the panoramic view takes in the Black Mountains to the east, including Mount Mitchell, and many of the peaks in the Great Smokies to the west. Walnut and Bluff Mountains do not offer any views, but the hike follows a beautiful wooded section of trail and crosses several small streams as it passes through the Roaring Fork Valley. Three shelters along this hike create several options for overnighting, but to divide the hike into two nearly equal days, you will need to use a tent. This hike gains less than 1,000 feet in elevation in the first 7 miles.

The Hike

From Max Patch Road, hike north on the A.T. and cross a creek before beginning the climb up the south slope of Max Patch. At mile 0.4, cross the gravel road and continue climbing Max Patch on steps cut into the side of the bald. Reach the summit (elevation 4,629 feet) in another 0.4 mile. Continue following the white-blazed post leading across the bald, and begin descending. In 0.4 mile, enter the woods.

At mile 2.2, cross Roaring Fork, and in 0.25 mile, reach an old railroad grade which the A.T. follows for 0.25 mile. The Trail crosses several small footbridges during the next 3 miles as you cross the northwest side of Roaring Fork Valley. At mile 5.8, reach a short side trail that leads to Roaring Fork Shelter. Water is available from a piped spring nearby. The privy offers a nice view of Roaring Fork Valley.

From the shelter, hike 0.5 mile to Lemon Gap, where the A.T. reaches, but does not cross, North Carolina 1182 (and Tennessee 107). In another 0.5 mile, begin climbing steadily up Walnut Mountain, and pass near the wooded summit (elevation 4,280 feet) at mile 7.3. In 0.25 mile, reach Walnut Mountain Shelter. Water is available from a somewhat unreliable spring near the shelter.

Continue north and descend, passing through fields on the way to Kale Gap in 0.75 mile. The Trail follows an old road bed for the next 0.25 mile and then passes around the side of Tennessee Bluff Mountain. The Trail passes through Catpen Gap in 0.75 mile and climbs to the wooded summit of Bluff Mountain (elevation 4,686 feet) at mile 9.9. During the remainder of the hike to Hot Springs, the A.T. loses well over 3,000 feet in elevation.

From Bluff Mountain, the Trail descends steadily for 3.7 miles to Garenflo Gap (elevation 2,500 feet) at mile 13.6. The Trail passes to the left of a forest service road in the gap. Continue north on the A.T., pass under power lines, turn right, and descend. Take a left 0.5 mile beyond Garenflo Gap and continue following the A.T. when you reach the junction with an old section of the A.T. that leads to right. The old A.T. rejoins the new path in 0.6 mile. Hike 1 mile, reach Little Bottom Gap, and climb a short steep section of trail. In another 1.3 miles, at mile 17, reach Gragg Gap. Deer Park Mountain Shelter is down a short side trail. Water is available from the small spring located between the A.T. and the shelter.

From Gragg Gap, climb Deer Park Mountain along the ridge. Reach a highpoint in about 1.5 miles and descend steadily into Hot Springs, North Carolina. During this descent, enjoy several good views of the town, particularly in the winter. At mile 19.9, reach the end of this hike.

Trailhead Directions

To get to Max Patch, the southern end of the hike, turn onto North Carolina 1175 from North Carolina 209, approximately 20 miles north of I-40 near Lake Junaluska and 7 miles south of Hot Springs, North Carolina. Follow NC 1175 for 5.3 miles and then turn onto Max Patch Road (North Carolina 1182). The parking area at the foot of the bald is 3 miles down Max Patch Road.

The northern trailhead is a forest service parking lot in Hot Springs, North Carolina. Hot Springs is 26 miles east of Newport, Tennessee and 17 miles northwest of Marshall, North Carolina, at the intersection of US 25/70 and NC 209. Inquire at the French Broad Ranger District Office on US 25/70 in Hot Springs for advice on parking.

MOUNT CAMMERER LOOP

great smoky mountains national park

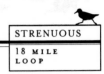

The highlight of this hike is the commanding panoramic view from the stone fire tower on the summit of Mount Cammerer. The mountain is the easternmost big peak in the park. Once known as White Rock, this peak was renamed for the former National Park Service Director, Arno Cammerer. Along this hike, you may witness some of the decline in the spruce-fir forest, caused in part by the balsam wooly adelgid. Acid rain is also believed to be a contributing factor in the demise of the trees because it makes mature fir easier prey for the adelgid.

This hike is set up with Cosby Knob Shelter as your overnight stop. Get a back-country permit in advance from Great Smoky Mountains National Park, Gatlinburg, Tennessee 37738, or call (865) 436-1231 for more information. The permits are free, but there is a fine for not obtaining one. In spite of this, you may want to bring a tent: illegal campers often fill up shelters before the hikers with permits arrive. We have had this happen more than once, and have had to sleep outside the shelter in our tent.

This strenuous hike should not be underestimated. The climbs and descents are quite difficult. There is a more than 3,000 feet difference in elevation between Davenport Gap and the fire tower on Cammerer.

THE HIKE

From the Trailhead at the Big Creek Ranger station, follow the Chestnut Branch Trail as it ascends gradually alongside Chestnut Branch for the first mile. The Trail then turns right and climbs steadily to its junction with the A.T. at mile 2 of the hike. Turn left and follow the white-blazed A.T. as it climbs Cammerer Ridge. At mile 2.9, pass the junction with the Lower Mount Cammerer Trail.

The A.T. climbs, often sharply, up the ridge. At mile 5.3, reach a side trail to the right that leads 0.6 mile to the summit of Mount Cammerer (elevation 5,025 feet). Turn right and follow the side trail up the ridge. After enjoying the tremendous view from the stone fire tower, return to the A.T. and continue hiking north as the Trail climbs for another 0.25 mile. (All hike mileages include the 1.2 round-trip to the fire tower) In 1.3 miles, (mile 8), cross the top of Rocky Face Mountain and descend 0.6 mile to Low Gap.

Begin climbing Cosby Knob, and in 0.75 mile, reach Cosby Knob Shelter just to the left of the A.T. Water is available from a nearby spring. After spending the night at the shelter, hike south on the A.T. for 0.75 mile to Low Gap. Turn right on Low Gap Trail, and descend steeply off the ridge as you follow Low Gap Branch down to Walnut

Bottoms. In 2.5 miles, reach the junction with the Big Creek Trail. Turn left and follow that trail on a gravel road as it winds alongside Big Creek for 5 miles. At the Big Creek Primitive Campground, turn left and walk 0.5 mile down the road to the Big Creek Ranger Station, the end of this hike.

TRAILHEAD DIRECTIONS

From I-40, take Exit 451 (Waterville) and follow North Carolina 284 south. The Big Creek Ranger Station is just past the village of Mount Sterling on NC 284.

MOUNT COLLINS AND CLINGMANS DOME

great smoky mountains national park

MODERATE

21.6 MILES
ROUND-TRIP

This overnight hike will take you over the highest point on the A.T. Clingmans Dome (elevation 6,643 feet). On clear days, there are outstanding views of the peaks of the Great Smokies from the observation tower. Formerly Smoky Dome, the peak is named after Thomas L. Clingman, a Civil War General and U.S. Senator. Clingman was known for his heated debate with Elisha Mitchell. The two argued over which peak in the state was the highest—Grandfather Mountain or Balsam Mountain. The debate took place through editorials in rival Asheville, North Carolina, newspapers. Mitchell died in a fall while trying to prove his claim that Balsam Mountain was the tallest. History proved Mitchell right, however, and the highest peak east of the Mississippi bears his name.

Another interesting site is found in Indian Gap, where an old roadbed crosses the Trail. It was built during the Civil War to get saltpeter mined from Alum Bluff Cave over the mountain to supply Confederate troops with gunpowder.

It is a round-trip hike from Newfound Gap to Double Springs Shelter. You will need to get a backcountry permit in advance from Great Smoky Mountains National Park, Gatlinburg, Tennessee 37738, or call (865) 436-1231 for more information. The permits are free, but there is a fine for not obtaining one. In spite of this, you may want to bring a tent: illegal campers often fill up shelters before the hikers with permits arrive. We have had this happen more than once, and have had to sleep outside the shelter in our tent.

Along this hike, you may witness some of the decline in the spruce-fir forest caused in part by the balsam wooly adelgid. Acid rain is also believed to be a contributing factor in the trees' demise as it makes mature fir easier prey for the adelgid.

THE HIKE

From the Trailhead at Newfound Gap, hike south on the A.T. Pass through a gap in the guardrail, and enter the woods. In 0.9 mile, pass the junction with the former A.T. on the left, and begin climbing along the southeast slope of Mount Mingus. In 0.25 mile, reach a highpoint on the side of Mount Mingus, and continue for 0.5 mile to Indian Gap. In the gap, you will also see the road to Clingmans Dome, which the Trail parallels but usually cannot be seen.

From Indian Gap, the A.T. climbs the ridge on the North Carolina–Tennessee state line, and reaches Little Indian Gap in 0.5 mile. In 1.9 miles, pass the junction with the Fork Ridge Trail on the left, at mile 4.1 of the hike. In another 0.4 mile, pass the junction with the Sugarland Mountain Trail on the right. The Mount Collins Shelter is 0.5 mile down this trail. Water is available from a nearby spring.

At mile 5, pass over the wooded summit of Mount Collins (elevation 6,188 feet), and begin a gentle descent on its southwest slope. In 0.6 mile, reach Collins Gap, then climb 1.1 miles to the tree-covered summit of Mount Love (elevation 6,446 feet). From Mount Love, descend to a sag on the eastern slope of Clingmans Dome, and climb steeply.

At mile 7.9, reach the Trail's highpoint on Clingmans Dome. A short side trail leads to the observation tower on the summit, which offers spectacular views on clear days. Unfortunately, the summit is often covered in clouds.

After returning to the A.T., continue hiking south and descend for 0.4 mile to a trail junction with Clingmans bypass trail. Continue following the A.T. and climb for. 1 mile to the summit of Mount Buckley (elevation 6,582 feet). From Buckley, the Trail descends sharply and then more gradually. Pass the junction with the Goshen Prong Trail at mile 10.2, and arrive at Double Springs Shelter at mile 10.8.

The shelter gets its name from springs located on both the North Carolina and the Tennessee side of the ridge. Bears are often seen in this area, so it's a good idea to use necessary precautions.

The return hike is north on the A.T. Hiking north from the shelter, reach the highpoint on Clingmans Dome in 2.9 miles, Mount Collins in another 2.9 miles, and Newfound Gap is 5 miles beyond Collins.

TRAILHEAD DIRECTIONS

Newfound Gap is on US 441 at the North Carolina–Tennessee state line, 16 miles south of Gatlinburg, Tennessee, and 20 miles north of Cherokee, North Carolina. There is ample parking in the gap.

RUSSELL FIELD, SPENCE FIELD, AND ROCKY TOP LOOP

great smoky mountains national park

STRENUOUS

14.7 MILES
ROUND-TRIP

This hike features a loop through Russell and Spence Fields to the bald summit of Rocky Top. Although it only uses 5 miles of the A.T., it is a spectacular overnight hike.

The hike begins at Cades Cove on the Tennessee side of the Smoky Mountains. You can pick up a map of the area at the ranger station. The loop follows the Anthony Creek Trail to the Russell Field Trail. At Russell Field, you pick up the A.T. to Spence Field and Rocky Top. Return by way of the A.T. to Spence Field, where you will pick up the Bote Mountain Trail, then follow it back to the Anthony Creek Trail.

Because you will stay at either Russell Field or Spence Field, you will need to get a backcountry permit in advance from Great Smoky Mountains National Park, Gatlinburg, Tennessee 37738, or call (865) 436-1231 for more information. The permits are free, but there is a fine for not obtaining one. In spite of this, you may want to bring a tent: illegal campers often fill up shelters before the hikers with permits arrive. We have had this happen more than once, and have had to sleep outside the shelter in our tent.

Along this hike, you may witness some of the decline in the spruce-fir forest caused in part by the balsam wooly adelgid. Acid rain is also believed to be a contributing factor in the trees demise as it makes mature fir easier prey for the adelgid.

THE HIKE

Starting from Cades Cove, follow the Anthony Creek Trail. You will follow this trail for 1.3 miles, mostly along a graded, gravel bed through a hardwood forest. The Trail follows and crisscrosses Anthony Creek, which makes for a pleasant walk.

At mile 1.3, turn right onto the Russell Field Trail, which at first follows the right prong of Anthony Creek through a hemlock and rhododendron forest. The growth is so thick and moss-covered here that it is very nearly tropical in appearance. From the right prong of Anthony Creek, the Trail follows Leadbetter Ridge for 1 mile, passes through a virgin hardwood forest in 0.5 mile, and crosses a grassy ridge in another 0.5 mile. Reach Russell Field and shelter at mile 4.8, 3.5 miles after turning onto Russell Field Trail. Water is available a short distance down the Russell Field Trail (toward Cades Cove).

From the shelter, turn left (north) onto the A.T. and hike just over 0.25 mile to McCampbell Gap (elevation 4,328 feet). Just over a mile later, reach the edge of the meadow at Little Bald, and enjoy excellent views to the south. Turn left, hike a short distance, and leave the meadow. Then turn right and enter the woods.

Follow the crest of the ridge through open woods, descend slightly, and reach

Spence Field at mile 6.4. Spence Field is often considered the western end of Thunderhead, the magnificent bald visible ahead. From the edge of this grassy field, it is just over a mile (2.6 miles total from Russell Field) to Spence Field Shelter.

At mile 7.4, reach the junction with the Eagle Creek Trail. It is a short distance down this trail to the shelter. The tributary of Eagle Creek is the Spence Cabin Branch of Gunna Creek. Water is available from a spring on the Trail past the shelter.

Continue along the A.T. for 1.2 miles to the summit of Rocky Top. You will descend slightly for nearly 0.5 mile to a grassy sag, where the Jenkins Ridge Trail heads right 6 miles to the Lakeshore Trail at Pickens Gap. From the sag, begin to climb up the grassy slope to Rocky Top. From the summit of Rocky Top (elevation 5,441 feet) there are great views of Fontana Lake. The summit of Thunderhead (elevation 5,527 feet) is another 0.6 mile from Rocky Top. It is covered in rhododendrons and is particularly beautiful in mid to late June. The side trip would add an extra 1.2 miles to the hike (a total of 15.9 miles).

Return to Spence Field by hiking south on the A.T. The Bote Mountain Trail enters the A.T. from the right. Take the graded Bote Mountain Trail for 1.7 miles. The first 0.5 mile is through a beech and birch forest, and the next 0.5 mile is through hemlock. The last 0.75 mile, before you rejoin the Anthony Creek Trail, is through a laurel grove. Rejoining the Anthony Creek Trail, you will pass through hardwood forest for 3.2 miles on the moderate to strenuous descent to Cades Cove, the end of the hike.

TRAILHEAD DIRECTIONS

The Trailhead for the Anthony Creek Trail is located at the Cades Cove Ranger Station. Take US 321 from US 441 south of Gatlinburg and Pigeon Forge. From US 321, take Tennessee 73 to Laurel Creek Road and follow the signs to the Great Smoky Mountains and Cades Cove.

NORTHERN NANTAHALA TRAVERSE

STRENUOUS

21.4 MILES
TRAVERSE

This hike takes you over Wayah and Wesser Balds, where spectacular views are afforded from old fire tower platforms. From these two lookouts, you can see many major peaks of the Great Smokies, other peaks south into the Nantahalas of North Carolina, and some of the mountains of Georgia. There is also a tremendous view from "Jumpup" on the long descent into the Nantahala Gorge.

The hike can be cut short by 4 miles by driving the forest service road to the top of Wayah Bald at the start of the hike. You will forego the long slow climb up from Wayah Gap, but may also miss a profusion of flame azaleas, rhododendrons, and mountain laurel in mid to late June and other seasonal wildflowers.

This hike is listed as strenuous because of the knee-jarring descent from Wesser Bald down to the Nantahala River. This traverse is difficult to set up because of the distance (by road) between the Trailheads, but it is worth it.

The Hike

From the Trailhead at Wayah Crest (elevation 4,180 feet), cross Wayah Road and hike north on the A.T., beginning the long climb up from the gap. During the first mile, USFS 69 will often be visible to the left of the Trail. At mile 1.3, pass the junction with the blue-blazed Wilson Lick Trail, which leads 0.1 mile to the left to a historic ranger station. Continue climbing for 0.5 mile, and at the top of a short steep climb, cross USFS 69. The piped Rattlesnake Spring is located just to the right of the Trail on USFS 69.

Climb the steps up from the road and continue a graded ascent. Reach the junction with the yellow-blazed Bartram Trail in another 0.5 mile. There is a campsite on the right and Wine Spring is just ahead on the left side of the Trail. The Bartram Trail and the A.T. share the same footpath for the next 2.1 miles. Beyond the spring, the Trail follows an old road bed for 0.25 mile before turning left off the road.

Continue hiking on a sidehill trail, and cross another old road in 1.4 miles. In 0.25 mile, the Trail joins a paved path leading from a gravel parking area to the top of Wayah Bald. As the A.T. turns onto the pavement, there is a USFS pit toilet on the left of the Trail. At mile 4.2, reach the stone observation tower on the summit of Wayah Bald (elevation 5,342 feet). Follow the A.T. north off the summit for 0.25 mile to where the Bartram Trail turns right and the A.T. continues ahead.

Continue north on the A.T. and reach Licklog Gap in 2 miles. Climb out of the gap to a highpoint on the ridge, and descend to Burningtown Gap in the next 2.3 miles. The dirt road in the gap is North Carolina 1397.

The Trail climbs out of the gap and reaches Cold Spring Shelter in 1.2 miles (mile 9.9). Water is available from the spring that is immediately in front of the shelter. This makes a good spot to overnight in order to break up the hike. Another good spot with potential campsites lies 2.2 miles beyond at a spring on the Trail.

Hike north from the shelter and climb on the western slope of Copper Ridge Bald. As the Trail continues following the ridgeline, it passes below the summits of Tellico, Black, and Rocky Balds. At mile 13.5, reach Tellico Gap. The gravel road is North Carolina 1365. Climb 1.4 miles from the gap to the highpoint on Wesser Bald (elevation 4,627 feet). A short side trail leads to the summit, where there is an old fire tower. The forest service, with help from the Nantahala Hiking Club, added a platform to the tower frame in 1993, and the tower now offers a tremendous view.

From Wesser Bald, descend 0.7 mile and pass the blue-blazed Wesser Creek Trail. In another 0.1 mile reach the Wesser Bald Shelter, built in 1994 (Wesser Creek is the shelter's water source). The A.T. follows a rough up-and-down route for the next 1.6 miles over to Jumpup, a rocky outlook with an awesome view down to the Nantahala Gorge. From Jumpup, at mile 17.3, hike a tough 3.3 miles downhill to the A. Rufus Morgan Shelter. At mile 21.4, reach US 19 just across the highway from the Nantahala River. The Nantahala Outdoor Center is just to the left of the Trail along the highway.

Trailhead Directions

The southern trailhead at Wayah Crest is on North Carolina 1310 (locally known as Wayah Road), 12 miles east of Franklin, North Carolina. The northern trailhead on US 19 in Wesser, North Carolina, is 15 miles west of Bryson City and 38 miles north of Murphy.

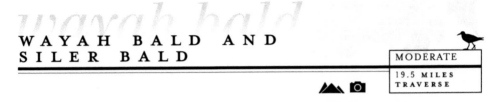

WAYAH BALD AND SILER BALD

MODERATE

19.5 MILES
TRAVERSE

This hike traverses two historic balds, both of which have been covered again in trees. From the top of Wayah Bald, there is, however, a tremendous view. Peaks from the Great Smokies south into Georgia can be viewed from the stone fire tower on the summit of Wayah.

The second bald, Siler Bald, though historically a bald, has also become covered once again with trees. Several years ago, the forest service cleared part of the summit and now maintains the meadow on Siler as a bald.

THE HIKE

From the Trailhead in Winding Stair Gap, cross the highway from the parking area, and hike north on the A.T. Climb up the slope by the road, and turn left to enter the woods. At mile 0.4, and again at mile 1, cross small streams as the Trail climbs to Panther Gap at mile 2.1. From that gap, descend for 0.5 mile and then begin climbing on the southeast slope of Siler Bald.

At mile 3.8, pass the junction with the blue-blazed Siler Bald Shelter Loop Trail, which turns off to the right 0.5 mile to the shelter and another 0.6 mile to rejoin the A.T. at mile 4.3. At the northern junction with the Loop Trail, a second trail leads 0.25 mile to the left to the cleared summit of Siler Bald (elevation 5,216 feet). The bald boasts fine views of the surrounding Nantahala Mountains. Wine Spring Bald with the radio towers and Wayah Bald with its stone tower can be seen to the northwest and north.

From the side trails to the summit and shelter, hike 1.7 miles down to Wayah Gap. The Wayah Crest Picnic Area is just to the left of the Trail, right before you get to North Carolina 1310 in the gap. Cross the highway (locally known as Wayah Road), and hike north on the A.T. Begin the long climb up from the gap. During the first mile of the hike, USFS 69 will often be visible to the left of the Trail. At mile 1.3, pass the junction with the blue-blazed Wilson Lick Trail, which leads 0.1 mile to the left to a historic ranger station. Continue climbing for 0.5 mile, and at the top of a short steep climb, cross USFS 69. The piped Rattlesnake Spring is located just to the right of the Trail on USFS 69.

Climb the steps up from the road and continue a graded ascent. Reach the junction with the yellow-blazed Bartram Trail in another 0.5 mile. There is a campsite on the right, and Wine Spring is just ahead on the left side of the Trail. The Bartram Trail and the A.T. share the same footpath for the next 2.1 miles. Beyond the spring, the Trail follows an old road bed for 0.25 mile before turning left off the road.

Continue hiking on a sidehill trail, and cross another old road in 1.4 miles. In 0.25 mile, the Trail joins a paved path leading from a gravel parking area to the top of Wayah Bald. As the A.T. turns onto the pavement, there is a USFS pit toilet on the left of the Trail. At mile 10.2, reach the stone observation tower on the summit of Wayah Bald (elevation 5,342 feet). Follow the A.T. north off the summit for 0.25 mile to where the Bartram Trail turns right and the white-blazed A.T. continues ahead.

Continue north on the A.T. and reach Licklog Gap in 2 miles. Climb out of the gap to a highpoint on the ridge, and descend to Burningtown Gap in the next 2.3 miles. The dirt road in the gap is North Carolina 1397. The Trail climbs out of the gap and reaches Cold Spring Shelter in 1.2 miles (mile 15.9). Water is available from the spring immediately in front of the shelter. In 2.2 miles, reach another spring on the Trail with possible campsites nearby.

Hike north from the shelter and climb on the western slope of Copper Ridge Bald. As the Trail continues following the ridgeline, it passes below the summits of Tellico, Black, and Rocky Balds. At mile 19.5, reach Tellico Gap, the northern end of the hike.

TRAILHEAD DIRECTIONS

The southern trailhead at Winding Stair Gap is on US 64, 10 miles east of Franklin, North Carolina. The northern trailhead is on gravel North Carolina 1365 in Tellico Gap. Take NC 1310 from US 19 in Beechertown, North Carolina. Drive a little over 5 miles from US 19, and follow NC 1365 when it turns to the left. Then drive 4 miles alongside Otter Creek to Tellico Gap.

STANDING INDIAN LOOP

STRENUOUS

25.4 MILES
LOOP

On this loop, you will be hiking through the Nantahala and Blue Ridge Mountains. A short side trail leads to Standing Indian (elevation 5,498 feet), which is the A.T.'s highest point south of the Smoky Mountains. From the summit, you can see the mountain ranges that the A.T. follows south to Springer Mountain (the southern terminus of the A.T.).

Albert Mountain is another highlight of this hike. Boasting one of the few remaining fire towers in the south, Albert affords spectacular views of the Blue Ridge and the Little Tennessee River Valley.

THE HIKE

This hike begins at Deep Gap (elevation 4,341 feet). Follow the A.T. south and immediately begin your ascent of Standing Indian Mountain. Note the blue-blazed Kimsey Creek Trail to your left. You will later take this 3.7-mile trail from Standing Indian Campground to complete your hike. From Deep Gap, it is 0.9 mile to a short side-trail leading to the Standing Indian Shelter.

The A.T. continues ahead, ascending along an old road. In another 1.5 miles or so, you will pass an unmarked trail on your left that leads to a spring. A short distance farther, you will reach the junction with the blue-blazed Lower Ridge Trail, which heads 0.1 mile to the summit of Standing Indian (to your right). To the left, the side trail heads 4.2 miles to Standing Indian Campground.

At mile 5.3, arrive at Beech Gap, where there are campsites and an intermittent spring to the right of the Trail. The blue-blazed Beech Gap Trail heads 2.8 miles to USFS 67, 4 miles south of Standing Indian Campground. Continue along the Trail and cross a number of streams in the next mile. Hike another 1.8 miles to Coleman Gap, located in a thick growth of rhododendrons.

In another mile, reach the junction with the blue-blazed Timber Ridge Trail to your left. This trail heads 2.3 miles to USFS 67, 4.4 miles south of Standing Indian Campground. Hike nearly 0.5 mile and reach Carter Gap at mile 8.5. Campsites and a shelter are a short distance to the left on a blue-blazed trail. Water is available from a spring located just beyond the shelter.

At mile 9.9, the A.T. heads left onto Little Ridgepole Mountain. This is where the A.T. leaves the Blue Ridge for the Nantahala Mountains. In just over 0.25 mile, reach the junction with an unmarked trail to your right that heads a short distance to good views. Hike another 2 miles to Betty Creek Gap (more campsites). A blue-blazed trail to your left heads 0.25 mile to a stream and USFS 67, 6.3 miles south of Standing Indian Campground.

The A.T. crosses the clearing and passes through a thick rhododendron growth. Nearly a mile later, the Trail reaches Mooney Gap and crosses USFS 83. To the right, this road heads to the Coweeta Hydrologic Laboratory and US 441. To the left, it joins USFS 67. From Deep Gap to Mooney Gap, the A.T. has been traveling through the Southern Nantahala Wilderness Area. At Mooney Gap, the Trail leaves the wilderness area, and in 0.1 mile, the Trail crosses a culvert that diverts water from the spring above the Trail.

Turn left, climb log steps, and leave the old road for a footpath. In another 0.25 mile, pass a cliff on Big Butt Mountain, and enjoy views of the Coweeta Valley. Hike just under 0.5 mile to Bearpen Gap where the A.T. passes near USFS 67.

At mile 14.4, reach the junction with two blue-blazed trails to your left. The Bear Pen Trail heads left across USFS 67 and descends 2.5 miles to join USFS 67 in the valley. The Albert Mountain Bypass Trail heads right, following the road around the mountain. The A.T. continues up Albert Mountain, a rocky 0.25-mile climb.

The summit of Albert (elevation 5,250 feet) has a fire tower that offers great views. The Trail then descends Albert for 0.25 mile and reaches the junction of the bypass trail to the left. A good spring is located several hundred yards down the bypass trail. Continue along the A.T. for another 0.4 mile to Big Spring Gap and the convergence of a number of trails. The blue-blazed trail to the left heads a short distance to Big Spring Shelter (mile 15.3). Water is available just beyond the shelter on the same trail.

The blue-blazed trail to the right is the Little Pinnacle Trail, which descends to Coweeta. The other trail to the right heads 0.25 mile to an outlook on Pinnacle Mountain. The A.T. continues to the left, crossing a stream in a boggy area in 2 miles.

Less than 0.5 mile after crossing the stream, reach Glassmine Gap, where the blue-blazed Long Branch Trail heads 2.3 miles to USFS 67 near Standing Indian Campground. One mile later, pass an intermittent spring to the left of the Trail. During the next mile, you will pass several potential campsites and intermittent water sources.

At mile 20.6, reach the blue-blazed trail that heads left to Rock Gap Shelter. Water is available from two springs just beyond and behind the shelter. In another 0.1 mile, pass the parking area at Rock Gap. Turn left on paved USFS 67 and hike one mile to Standing Indian Campground, where you will pick up the Kimsey Creek Trail. At Rock Gap, USFS 67 heads right 0.5 mile to Wallace Gap. The blue-blazed trail on the right leads 0.75 mile to the huge John Wasilik Memorial Poplar.

Pick up the Kimsey Creek Trail at Standing Indian Campground, and follow Kimsey Creek 3.7 miles back to Deep Gap. The Trail begins at the Backcountry Information Center and crosses the river on the campground road before turning right and following the edge of the campground. In just over 0.25 mile, the Kimsey Creek Trail turns left and leaves the Trails that follow the river. About 0.5 mile later, the Trail enters a clearing and turns right along a gated road that follows the creek.

At mile 23.8, cross a log bridge over another creek, and at mile 25.4, reach Deep Gap by way of the former picnic and camping area.

Trailhead Directions

Reach Deep Gap by taking USFS 71 from US 64 (south of Franklin, North Carolina) near the Clay–Macon county line. The road is to the left if you are coming from Franklin. Drive 6 miles on USFS 71 to Deep Gap.

GEORGIA IS THE LAST STATE ON THE TRAIL
(OR THE FIRST FOR MOST THRU-HIKERS). ITS MORE
THAN 75 MILES OF TRAIL ARE EXTREMELY POPULAR
YEAR-ROUND. THE TRAIL TRAVERSES THE
CHATTAHOOCHEE NATIONAL FOREST AND IS
NOTED FOR ITS RUGGED WILDERNESS AREAS AND HIGH
ELEVATIONS. POPULAR HIKING SPOTS INCLUDE THE
SWAG OF THE BLUE RIDGE, TRAY MOUNTAIN,
ROCKY MOUNTAIN, BLUE MOUNTAIN,

Georgia

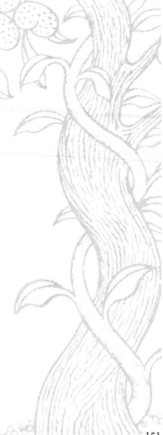

WOLF LAUREL TOP, BLOOD MOUNTAIN, AND
BIG CEDAR MOUNTAIN. NEELS GAP, AT THE BASE
OF BLOOD MOUNTAIN, OFFERS THE WALASI-YI
MOUNTAIN CROSSINGS STORE. IT IS THE ONLY BUILD-
ING THROUGH WHICH THE A.T. PASSES. SPRINGER
MOUNTAIN IS THE SOUTHERN TERMINUS OF THE A.T.
A BRONZE PLAQUE CREATED BY THE
GEORGIA APPALACHIAN TRAIL CLUB
MARKS THE MOUNTAIN AS THE
SOUTHERN TERMINUS OF THE A.T.

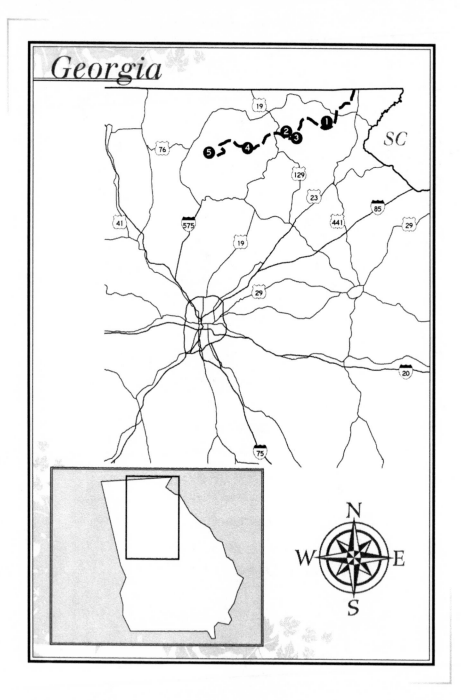

Georgia

SC

1. TRAY MOUNTAIN WILDERNESS
2. WOLF LAUREL TOP AND BLOOD MOUNTAIN
3. BLOOD MOUNTAIN LOOP
4. WOODY GAP AND SPRINGER MOUNTAIN
5. SPRINGER MOUNTAIN AND THREE FORKS LOOP

TRAY MOUNTAIN
WILDERNESS

This short overnight hike crosses some of the biggest mountains on the Georgia section of the A.T. and has several long gap-to-mountain ascents. During the 6.4-mile section from Addis Gap to Tray Gap, you will hike through the heart of the Tray Mountain Wilderness Area. You will also cross the rocky summit of Tray Mountain, which offers tremendous views of the surrounding mountains from the foothills in the south to the Nantahala Mountains in North Carolina. Though there are a few tough climbs and descents, this hike is listed as moderate, in part, because it is only 16.1 miles long.

THE HIKE

From Dicks Creek Gap, hike south on the A.T., follow the road briefly, and turn left to enter the woods. Climb up out of the gap, cross several creeks, and reach Moreland Gap at mile 1.2. Climb 1 mile to the top of Powell Mountain (elevation 3,850 feet). Descend 0.25 mile to McClure Gap, climb, then descend along the ridge, and reach Deep Gap 1.1 miles later. A 0.25-mile blue-blazed trail leads to Deep Gap Shelter. Water is available from the spring you pass on the way to the shelter.

Climb up from Deep Gap, reaching a highpoint on Kelly Knob (the Trail does not cross the summit) at mile 4.2. Descend 1.1 miles to Addis Gap. Some old guidebooks mention an Addis Gap Shelter, which has

been removed. From Addis Gap, climb 0.6 mile to a highpoint on the ridge and descend 0.25 mile to Sassafras Gap at mile 6. 1.

Cross over the east side of Round Top, and traverse the broad gap known as the Swag of the Blue Ridge (elevation 3,400 feet), about a mile beyond Sassafras Gap. Climb up from the Swag and pass around the western slope of Young Lick Knob. Descend to Steeltrap Gap at mile 8.9. The Appalachian Trail Guide to North Carolina-Georgia states that water is available to the left of the Trail in this gap.

Ascend and then descend on the ridge during the 1.5 miles to Wolfpen Gap. Begin climbing on the eastern slope of Tray Mountain. In 1.2 miles, at mile 10.6, reach the junction with a blue-blazed side trail that leads 0.25 mile to the right to Tray Mountain Shelter. Water is available from a piped spring on a blue-blazed trail a short distance behind the shelter. Although it does not break the hike up into two equal sections, we suggest you camp here. It is a nice place to camp whether you stay in the shelter or not, and there is easy access to water.

After passing the shelter side trail, continue to climb, sometimes steeply, for 0.25 mile to the rocky summit of Tray Mountain (elevation 4,430 feet). Enjoy a spectacular view from the peak. Descend on switchbacks to Tray Gap at mile 11.7, cross the dirt USFS 79 in the gap, and enter the woods beside the small parking area. Descend, crossing USFS 79 again in 1 mile, and reach

Indian Grave Gap and a dirt forest service road in another 0.75 mile. A blue-blazed bypass trail leads to the right (down the road) and rejoins the A.T. in 2.5 miles on the other side of Rocky Mountain.

After crossing the dirt road, climb the eastern slope of Rocky Mountain, reaching the summit (elevation 4,017 feet) at mile 14.8. Descend steadily from Rocky Mountain, and in 0.25 mile, pass the junction with the blue-blazed bypass trail that leads back to Indian Grave Gap. In another 0.25 mile, cross a tributary of the Hiawasee River, and 0.6 mile later, reach the southern end of the hike in Unicoi Gap.

TRAILHEAD DIRECTIONS

Dicks Creek Gap is on US 76, 11 miles east of Hiawasee. The southern trailhead at Unicoi Gap is on Georgia 75, 9 miles north of Helen.

WOLF LAUREL TOP AND BLOOD MOUNTAIN

MODERATE

15.8 MILES
TRAVERSE

Good views and the highest peak on the A.T. in Georgia are the highlights of this relatively short overnight hike. On this section, the A.T. passes good viewpoints on Cowrock and Wolf Laurel Top Mountains, and climbs up to Blood Mountain to offer another spectacular view. There is also a fine view from Big Cedar Mountain.

The nearly 11 miles from Neels Gap to Woody Gap attract more visitors than any other section of the A.T. in Georgia. The biggest attraction, Blood Mountain, was named after a battle between the Creek and Cherokee Indians that caused the mountain to run red with blood.

At Neels Gap you will pass under the arch at the Walasi-Yi Center, which is the only covered section on the entire A.T. The center's name is Indian for Frogtown; and Neels Gap was once known as Frogtown Gap. The center has a good selection of books, backpacking equipment, food, and more. This is a tough hike that is listed as moderate because it is only 16 miles long.

THE HIKE

From the trailhead in Tesnatee Gap, hike south on the A.T. and climb steadily for 0.75 mile to the top of Cowrock Mountain (elevation 3,842 feet). Enjoy a fine view from the rocks just before the summit and another fine view from the campsite to the left of the Trail on the summit. Descend to a sag and then climb Wolf Laurel Top, reaching the summit (elevation 3,766 feet) at mile 2.1, where there is a good viewpoint on the rocks to the left of the Trail. Descend and follow the ridge, pass below the summits of Rock Spring Top and Turkeypen Mountain, and reach Swaim Gap at mile 3.4.

Climb Levelland Mountain on switchbacks, and reach the summit (elevation 3,942 feet) 0.6 mile from Swaim Gap. Descend from Levelland, and in 1.5 miles, pass under the arch at the Walasi-Yi Center in Neels Gap, which is the only covered section on the entire A.T. If you would like to camp on Blood Mountain, you will want to carry your water up from here because there is no water on the summit.

In Neels Gap (elevation 3,125 feet), cross US 19/129 and enter the woods. After crossing the road, look on the right side of the Trail at the base of the steps for the brass plaque set in the rock that is identical to the one at the southern terminus of the Trail on Springer Mountain. In 0.9 mile, pass the blue-blazed trail on the right that leads 0.25 mile to a parking area for day hikers. Shortly thereafter, the Trail begins to climb Blood Mountain in earnest. The steady 1.4-mile climb is generally well-graded on switchbacks. There are a couple of excellent views from the Trail near the top of the climb as well as from the rocks over the shelter on the summit (elevation 4,461 feet). The two-room stone cabin was built by the CCC in the 1930s. At mile 7.9, the summit makes a good place to spend the night, leaving 8.3 miles for the second day.

Descend steeply from Blood Mountain on a mostly gentle path, with stone steps provided in the steep sections, and reach Slaughter Creek Spring in 0.5 mile. Tent sites are available near the spring. In the next 0.25 mile, cross two small creeks and reach Bird Gap at mile 9.9. Pass a blue-blazed trail on the left that leads around Blood Mountain. Climb out of the gap on the side of Turkey Stamp Mountain and then descend to Horsebone Gap. Climb up from that gap on the side of Gaddis Mountain, and descend to Jarrard Gap at mile 10.9.

In Jarrard Gap, pass a blue-blazed trail on the right that leads down to Lake Winfield Scott, and climb 0.5 mile to a highpoint on Burnett Field Mountain (elevation 3,478 feet). In another 1.2 miles, pass the Dockery Lake Trail and begin climbing Granny Top Mountain, reaching the summit at mile 14.

Descend Granny Top, and in 0.25 mile, begin the 1-mile climb up Big Cedar Mountain (elevation 3,737 feet). There are fine views from the rocks near the top of the mountain. Big Cedar is referred to as Preaching Rock on the Chattahoochee National Forest Map. Descend sharply for 0.25 mile from Big Cedar to Lunsford Gap. From that gap, climb slightly and then descend to Woody Gap at mile 16.2, the end of the hike.

TRAILHEAD DIRECTIONS

From Helen, drive north on Georgia 75 to Georgia 356. From GA 356, drive to Georgia 348 and turn right. Drive about 12 miles from the town of Helen to the trailhead in Tesnatee Gap.

Woody Gap is on US 60 at a point 5.6 miles north of Stone Pile Gap, which is about 9 miles north of Dahlonega on US 19. There is a picnic area at the trailhead.

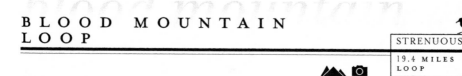

BLOOD MOUNTAIN LOOP

STRENUOUS

19.4 MILES
LOOP

This loop hike uses the A.T., the Slaughter Creek Trail, Coosa Backcountry Trail, Jarrard Gap Trail and a very short section of the Duncan Ridge Trail to loop through the north Georgia mountains.

The major feature of this hike is Blood Mountain, the highest peak on the A.T. in Georgia. The mountain takes its name from a battle between the Creek and Cherokee Indians that caused the mountain to run red with blood. There is an excellent view the shelter on the summit (elevation 4,461 feet) of Blood Mountain. The two-room stone cabin was built by the Civilian Conservation Corps in the 1930s. Please note that the hub of this loop was once Slaughter Gap. The Georgia Appalachian Trail Club undertook an extensive series of trail relocations in early 2004 to move the trails out of the over-impacted Slaughter Gap. Please do not camp in that gap as the GATC is trying to restore its wilderness character.

THE HIKE

From the trailhead at Lake Winfield Scott, the Slaughter Creek and Jarrard Gap Trails share the same path for the 0.25 mile. Take the Slaughter Creek Trail, which ascends to the slopes above the stream. At mile 1.7 of the hike, the Trail follows a logging road along Slaughter Creek. Cross Slaughter Creek for the last time at mile 2.2. Ascend for 0.5 mile to Slaughter Gap, and a junction with the A.T.

From here, the summit of Blood Mountain is 0.5 mile north on the white-blazed A.T. After taking in the view from the summit, which is best seen from the rock ledge overshadowing the stone shelter, descend on the A.T. and in 0.25 mile take the blue-blazed Duncan Ridge Trail.

Follow the blue-blazed Duncan Ridge Trail, to its junction with yellow-blazed Coosa Backcountry Trail (C.B.T.). Turn right and continue hiking on the C.B.T., which switchbacks through the fern-filled forest as it descends nearly 2,000 feet in elevation to Vogel State Park. Beginning at mile 4.7, the C.B.T. shares the path with the Bear Hair Gap Trail for the last 1.4 miles down to the park, where the trail briefly follows a park road.

Continue hiking the C.B.T., turning right off the road, cross Burnett Branch and ascend to Georgia 180 in Burnett Gap (elevation 2,800 feet) at mile 7.1 of the hike. Turn right on an old road, descending to the West Fork of Wolf Creek at mile 9.4. Cross the creek on the log bridge. The trail then turns right on USFS 107 before turning left into the woods.

Ascend Ben Knob to Locust Stake Gap (elevation 2,540 feet) at mile 10.7 of the hike. Continue ascending to Calf Stomp in another 1.4 miles. After crossing Calf Stomp Road, the C.B.T. ascends on a strenuous climb to Coosa Bald, gaining 1,060 feet in elevation in just over one mile. A quarter mile into this ascent you will cross a small stream, which is the last water source for the next 3.8 miles.

At mile 13.1, reach a high point on Coosa Bald and shortly after, the junction with the Duncan Ridge Trail (the summit of Coosa Bald is .2 mile to the right on the Duncan Ridge Trail). Turn left, following the C.B.T. and Duncan Ridge Trail as they descend from the Bald. In .5 mile, the trail turns left onto USFS 39, which it follows briefly, before turning back into the woods. From there the trail ascends to Wildcat Knob at mile 13.9 of the hike.

The trail descends for .6 mile to GA 180 in Wolfpen Gap (elevation 3,260 feet). Cross the road and climb .9 mile to Slaughter Mountain (4,140 feet). It is a relatively easy 0.7 mile back to the point where this hike began its loop on the Coosa Backcountry Trail. Continue straight along the blue-blazed Duncan Ridge Trail the 0.2 mile to the junction with the A.T. and turn right hiking south toward Slaughter Creek Spring.

From Slaughter Creek Spring, continue following the white-blazed A.T. south, reaching Bird Gap in .5 mile and Jarrard Gap in another 1.4 miles. From Jarrard Gap, take the blue-blazed Jarrard Gap Trail descending 1.2 miles to Lake Winfield Scott and the end of this hike.

TRAILHEAD DIRECTIONS

From Dahlonega, drive about 9 miles north on US 19 to its junction with Georgia 60 in Stone Pile Gap. Continue north on GA 60 to the junction with GA 180 in Suches. Turn right, heading east on GA 180 for just under 4.5 miles. Turn right on Lake Winfield Scott Road. The trailhead sign and parking area are at the south end of the lake (just beyond the bridge).

WOODY GAP AND SPRINGER MOUNTAIN

MODERATE
20.9 MILES TRAVERSE

The first 12 miles of this traverse follow long ridges as the A.T. winds its way toward the southern terminus of the A.T.— Springer Mountain. Along the way, the Trail skirts the 3,742-foot Black Mountain near Woody Gap, and from Hightower Gap, it is just 8 miles to the summit of Springer.

At Three Forks, three mountain streams join to form Noontootla Creek. The Trail then follows Stover Creek through one of the highlights of this hike—a stand of virgin hemlocks known as the Cathedral Hemlocks. Hiking north from Springer, you won't see trees like this again until the Great Smoky Mountains.

THE HIKE

From Woody Gap (elevation 3,050 feet), cross through a picnic area and begin your ascent along Black Mountain. You will climb, then descend to Tritt Gap (elevation 3,050 feet) in the next mile. From Tritt Gap, hike just under 0.5 mile to the crest of Ramrock Mountain (elevation 3,200 feet) and enjoy nice views to the south. Descend along switchbacks for 0.1 mile to Jacks Gap (elevation 3,000 feet), and begin to climb again before descending to Liss Gap (elevation 2,952 feet) at mile 2.1.

At mile 2.6, cross an old road, begin to climb, reach the top of the ridge at mile 3, and then descend to Gooch Gap. Just before you reach the gap, you will pass a blue-blazed side trail to your left that heads a short distance to a spring. At mile 3.6, reach USFS 42 at Gooch Gap (elevation 2,784 feet). USFS 42 heads right 2.7 miles to Suches, and left 6.1 miles to Cooper Gap and (eventually) the base of Springer Mountain.

Shortly beyond USFS 42, reach the junction with another blue-blazed side trail, which forms a 0.25-mile loop back to the A.T. as it passes Gooch Gap Shelter. Water is available from a spring near the shelter sign at the southern approach to the loop. Continue along the A.T. for 0.25 mile to the southern end of the loop where the blue-blazed trail rejoins the A.T.

After passing the side trail, hike nearly another 0.75 mile to a gap (elevation 2,950 feet). Climb to the ridge top and reach the high point of Horseshoe Ridge at mile 5. Descend to the right, following a stream.

In nearly 0.5 mile, cross the stream, turn left at the bottom of the hill, and continue along the A.T. with former pastures to your right. Hike 0.75 mile to Blackwell Creek and cross on a footbridge. There are good campsites to your right. Continue along the A.T., ascend through rhododendrons, and cross another stream in 0.5 mile.

In 0.25 mile, cross Justus Creek on a footbridge (more campsites along the creek), and in another 0.1 mile, reach an old logging road. A left on this road will take you to Suches-Cooper Gap Road (USFS 42). Begin to climb Justus Mountain, reaching Phyllis Spur (elevation 3,081 feet) in 0.75 mile; descend into a sag (elevation 2,900 feet) 0.25 mile later, and reach the summit of Justus (elevation 3,224 feet) at mile 7.8. From the summit, head left along the ridge before descending along switchbacks.

In just over 0.5 mile, reach the intersection of three roads at Cooper Gap (elevation 2,828 feet). The road heading downhill to the left is Cooper Gap Road (USFS 80), which heads 14 miles to Dahlonega. To your left and ahead is USFS 42, which heads left back to Gooch Gap and Suches, and ahead to Springer Mountain. To your right is USFS 15, which heads to the small settlement of Gaddistown. Cross USFS 42 and begin an ascent up Sassafras Mountain.

Reach the summit (elevation 3,336 feet) at mile 9. As you descend off the ridge top, keep an eye out for U.S. Army Rangers who perform maneuvers in this area (often well into the night), which include automatic weapon fire. It is 1 mile from the summit of Sassafras to Horse Gap (elevation 2,673 feet). You should be able to see USFS 42 to your right. Climb the ridge again, hike along the ridge crest, and descend to Hightower Gap at mile 11.7.

Reach the intersection of USFS 42 in Hightower Gap (elevation 2,854 feet) at mile 11.9. To your right, USFS 42 heads back to Cooper Gap and Suches. Ahead, USFS 42 heads on to Winding Stair Gap and Springer Mountain. Between these two roads is USFS 69, which heads 2 miles to Rock Creek Lake. Continue along the A.T. and climb 0.5 mile, passing the 0.1 mile side trail to Hawk Mountain Shelter. Built in 1993, the post and beam shelter has a loft and can accommodate a number of hikers. Water is available from the stream downhill in front of the shelter.

The A.T. continues along the north side of Hawk Mountain. The Trail over the summit was abandoned in 1979. Reach the ridge crest and the intersection of the former A.T. in just over 0.5 mile. Begin to descend, and at mile 14.2, arrive at a logging road. Hickory Flats Cemetery Road heads left to USFS 58 near Three Forks. To reach the cemetery, hike a short distance down this road. At the left turn in the gravel road, take a right along a dirt road. There are picnic tables and a pavilion at the cemetery.

Continue along the A.T., cross the road, descend for just over 0.25 mile, and turn left onto an old logging road. In another 0.4 mile, reach the intersection of the Benton MacKaye Trail (white-diamond blazes) and Duncan Ridge Trail (blue blazes) to your right. The three trails (A.T. included) share the same footpath for the next mile.

In 0.1 mile, reach a blue-blazed side trail that heads right to Long Creek Falls, a pretty waterfall. As the A.T. parallels Long Creek, you will pass many possible campsites. At mile 15.9, reach USFS 58 at Three Forks. USFS 58 heads left 2.6 miles to Winding Stair Gap and USFS 42. The Duncan Ridge Trail ends here, but the Benton MacKaye continues to follow the A.T.'s path for a short distance before turning left up Rich Mountain. Cross the road, and soon thereafter, Chester Creek.

Hike 0.5 mile past Three Forks, and cross Stover Creek. Turn left, and follow an old logging road that parallels the creek. Here, the Trail passes through Cathedral Hemlocks, a virgin stand of timber. One mile later, turn left off the road and soon cross a bridge over a stream before climbing log steps. In 0.1 mile, reach another logging road. Stover Creek Shelter is to the right. The A.T. turns left and follows the road a short distance before ascending log steps to the right. At the top of the steps, reach another road, turn left, and follow it for 0.25 mile before ascending more steps to your right.

As you climb the north slope of Rich Mountain, cross a stream at mile 17.9 and reach the ridge top (and the intersection of the Benton MacKaye Trail) in just over 0.25 mile. Head right, continue to climb along Rich Mountain, and cross another old road in

just over 0.5 mile. The Benton MacKaye Trail leaves the A.T. here, but rejoins it on Springer Mountain. The old road heads left to a blue-blazed side trail that leads downhill to water.

At mile 19.1, reach the junction of USFS 42 just below Springer Mountain. Ascend along a relocated section of trail up Springer Mountain. At mile 19.8, reach the junction with the Benton MacKaye Trail where it leaves the A.T. for the first time after sharing its southern terminus with Springer. A short distance later, reach the blue-blazed side trail that leads to Springer Mountain Shelter. The mountain boasts a shelter, built in 1992, that accommodates more hikers than the earlier shelter and includes a sleeping loft. Water is available from a nearby spring.

The summit of Springer (elevation 3,782 feet) is reached at mile 20. To the left of the Trail is a bronze marker set into the rock marking this as the southern terminus of the Appalachian National Scenic Trail. The plaque, placed here in 1993, features a map of the Trail's route from Maine to Georgia. After passing this marker, the Trail turns to the right, where the southernmost blaze is painted on a rock outcropping with wonderful views of the Blue Ridge. A bronze plaque in this rock near the blaze features a backpacker and the words , "Appalachian Trail. Georgia to Maine. A footpath for those who seek fellowship with the wilderness. The Georgia Appalachian Trail Club." This marker was made in 1933 and placed here in 1959 by the Georgia club, when the southern terminus was moved from Mount Ogelthorpe to Springer Mountain because of encroaching development.

A blue-blazed trail heads 8.3 miles to Amicalola Falls State Park. Return to the base of Springer on USFS 42 (0.9 mile) to complete this overnight hike.

Woody Gap is on US 60 at a point 5.6 miles north of Stone Pile Gap, which is about 9 miles north of Dahlonega on US 19. There is a picnic area at the trailhead.

The parking area at Springer Mountain can be reached by taking GA 60 north from Woody Gap. Turn left on USFS 42, which is paved for the first several miles, and continue to the Trail crossing. You will cross the A.T. in Gooch, Cooper, and Hightower Gaps before reaching the trailhead near Springer. It is a long drive down USFS 42, but this road is often open when other forest service roads in the area are not.

SPRINGER MOUNTAIN AND THREE FORKS LOOP

MODERATE

10.1 MILES LOOP

This loop hike uses the A.T. and Benton MacKaye Trail (B.M.T.) figure eight between Springer Mountain and Three Forks. The hike will take you to two viewpoints along Springer Mountain, which is the southern terminus of both the A.T. and the B.M.T. The Benton MacKaye Trail is named for the man who provided the inspiration for the A.T. in a 1921 article for *The Journal of the American Institute of Architects*. The B.M.T. follows the more westerly route first proposed for the A.T. and was created to take some of the hiking pressure off the oft-hiked A.T. in Georgia.

THE HIKE

From the trailhead on USFS 42, hike south on the A.T. and begin the steady, gradual climb up Springer on a sidehill trail. At mile 0.75, reach the junction with the 0.25-mile side trail leading to Springer Mountain Shel-

ter. Hike another 0.25 mile to the southern terminus of the A.T. There is a trail register in a mailbox on a tree near the rock face. After visiting the summit of Springer, head back the direction you came traveling north on the A.T. for 0.2 mile to the turn off for the Benton MacKaye Trail.

Descend Springer on the B.M.T., which is blazed with white diamonds. In 1.2 mile, pass a sign marking a view to the right of the Trail. Continue along the B.M.T. for 0.3 mile to USFS 42 at Big Stamp Gap. Cross the Forest Service road and follow the Trail on gentle terrain until crossing an old road in a half mile at mile 3.2 of the hike. In 1 mile, join the A.T. The two trails share the same path along Rich Mountain for 0.6 mile. When the trails split, remain on the white-diamond-blazed B.M.T. and in 0.3 mile reach and follow an old woods road as the Trail descends. In 0.9 mile, at mile 6.9 of the hike, the B.M.T. rejoins the A.T. and the two trails descend together 0.1 mile to Three Forks, where Chester, Long, and Stover Creeks join to form Noontootla Creek.

Return, by going back the direction you came this time following the rectangular white blazes of the A.T. each time the two trails diverge. The Trail ascends along Stover Creek for about two miles. The trailhead at USFS 42 is 3.1 miles south on the A.T. from Three Forks.

Trailhead Directions

To get to this trail crossing, take USFS 42 from GA 60 just north of Woody Gap. From Dahlonega, drive about 9 miles north on US 19 to its junction with Georgia 60 in Stone Pile Gap. Go north about 5.5 miles on GA 60 to Woody Gap. There is parking and a picnic area at the trailhead. Just north of Woody Gap, turn left on USFS 42, which is paved for the first several miles, and continue to the Trail crossing. You will cross the A.T. in Gooch, Cooper, and Hightower Gaps before coming to the trailhead near Springer. This road is often open when USFS 28 and 77 are not.

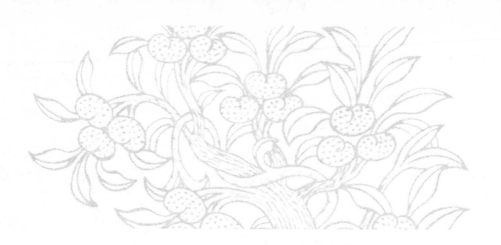

Appendix

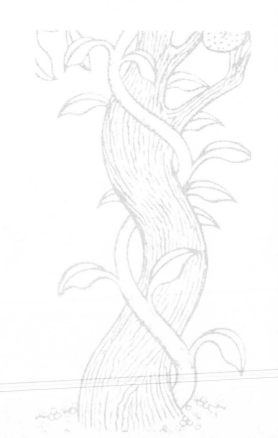

TRAIL MAINTENANCE CLUBS

The Appalachian Trail owes its existence to the hiking clubs, which are charged with its maintenance. These clubs are responsible not only for the maintenance of the footpath but also for relocating the trail, managing its surrounding lands, helping with land acquisition negotiations, compiling and updating guidebook and map information, working with trail communities on both problems and special events, and recruiting and training new maintainers.

The A.T. is maintained and protected by clubs and organizations along its length. If you are interested in local hikes or other activities in your area, check out the clubs and trail organizations near you.

Addresses appear for those with permanent offices or post office boxes. Occasionally these do change; in this case, please contact ATC headquarters for the address of the current club president or other appropriate officer (P. O. Box 807, Harpers Ferry, West Virginia 25425, or www.appalachiantrail.org).

GEORGIA, NORTH CAROLINA, AND TENNESSEE

GEORGIA APPALACHIAN TRAIL CLUB
P. O. Box 654, Atlanta, GA 30301
Voice mailbox: (404) 634-6495
www.georgia-atclub.org
Springer Mountain to Bly Gap, N.C.

NANTAHALA HIKING CLUB
173 Carl Slagle Road
Franklin, NC 28734
www.maconweb.com/nhc
Bly Gap, N.C. to Wesser, N.C.

SMOKY MOUNTAINS HIKING CLUB
P. O. Box 1454
Knoxville, TN 37901
www.esper.com/smhc
Wesser, N.C. to Davenport Gap

CAROLINA MOUNTAIN CLUB
P. O. Box 68
Asheville, NC 28802
www.carolinamtnclub.com
Davenport Gap to Spivey Gap, N.C.

TENNESSEE EASTMAN HIKING CLUB
P. O. Box 511
Kingsport, TN 37662
www.tehcc.org
Spivey Gap, N.C. to Damascus, VA

VIRGINIA, WEST VIRGINIA, AND MARYLAND

Mount Rogers Appalachian Trail Club
24198 Green Spring Road
Abingdon, VA 24211-5320
www.geocities.com/Yosemite/Geyser/253
Damascus, VA to VA 670

PIEDMONT APPALACHIAN TRAIL HIKERS
P. O. Box 4423
Greensboro, NC 27404
www.path-at.org
VA 670 to VA 623; VA 615 to VA 612

OUTDOOR CLUB OF VIRGINIA TECH
P. O. Box 538
Blacksburg, VA 24063
www.fbox.vt.edu/org/outdoor
VA 623 to VA 615; VA 612 to VA 611; US 460 to Pine Swamp Branch Shelter

ROANOKE APPALACHIAN TRAIL CLUB
P. O. Box 12282
Roanoke, VA 24024
www.ratc.org
VA 611 to US 460; Pine Swamp Branch Shelter to Black Horse Gap

NATURAL BRIDGE APPALACHIAN TRAIL CLUB
P. O. Box 3012
Lynchburg, VA 24503
www.nbatc.org
Black Horse Gap to Tye River

TIDEWATER APPALACHIAN TRAIL CLUB
P. O. Box 8246
Norfolk, VA 23503
www.tidewateratc.org
Tye River to Reeds Gap

OLD DOMINION APPALACHIAN TRAIL CLUB
P. O. Box 25283
Richmond, VA 23260
www.odatc.org
Reeds Gap to Rockfish Gap

POTOMAC APPALACHIAN TRAIL CLUB
118 Park Street SE
Vienna, VA 22180
(703) 242-0693
www.patc.net
Rockfish Gap, VA, to Pine Grove Furnace State Park, PA

PATC LOCAL CHAPTERS
CHARLOTTESVILLE CHAPTER
John Shannon (434) 293-2953

SOUTHERN SHENANDOAH VALLEY
CHAPTER
Michael Seth (540) 438-1301
Northern Shenandoah Valley Chapter
Lee Sheaffer (540) 955-0736
thumpers@visuallink.com

WEST VIRGINIA CHAPTER
Judy Smoot (540) 667-2036
wvpatc@hotmail.com
www.patc-wv.org

NORTH CHAPTER
Pete Brown (410) 343-1140
northchapter@patc.net
www.patc.net/chapters/north

PENNSYLVANIA
The Potomac Appalachian Trail Club also maintains the A.T. in Pennsylvania, from the Penn./Maryland state line to Pine Grove Furnace State Park.

MOUNTAIN CLUB OF MARYLAND
7923 Galloping Circle
Baltimore, MD 21244-1254
(410) 377-6266
www.mcomd.org
Pine Grove Furnace State Park, PA, to Center Point Knob; Darlington Trail to Susquehanna River

CUMBERLAND VALLEY APPALACHIAN TRAIL
CLUB
P. O. Box 395
Boiling Springs, PA 17007
www.geocities.com/cvatclub
Center Point Knob to Darlington Trail

YORK HIKING CLUB
2684 Forest Road
York, PA 17402
(717) 244-6769
www.angelfire.com/pa2/
yorkhikingclub/index.html
Susquehanna River to PA 225

SUSQUEHANNA APPALACHIAN TRAIL CLUB
Box 61001
Harrisburg, PA 17106-1001
www.libertynet.org/susqatc
PA 225 to Clarks Valley

BLUE MOUNTAIN EAGLE CLIMBING CLUB
P. O. Box 14982
Reading, PA 19612-4982
www.bmecc.org
Rausch Gap Shelter to Tri-County Corner;
Bake Oven Knob Road to Lehigh Furnace Gap

ALLENTOWN HIKING CLUB
P. O. Box 1542
Allentown, PA 18105-1542
www.allentownhikingclub.org
Tri-County Corner to Bake Oven Knob Road

PHILADELPHIA TRAIL CLUB
741 Golf Drive
Warrington, PA 18976
(215) 343-1695
www.m.zanger.tripod.com/index
Lehigh Furnace Gap to Little Gap

AMC-DELAWARE VALLEY CHAPTER
1180 Greenleaf Drive
Bethlehem, PA 18017-9319
www.amcdv.org
Little Gap to Wind Gap

BATONA HIKING CLUB
6651 Eastwood Street
Philadelphia, PA 19149-2331
members.aol.com/Batona
Wind Gap to Fox Gap

WILMINGTON TRAIL CLUB
P. O. Box 1184
Wilmington, DE 19899
www.wilmingtontrailclub.org
Fox Gap to Delaware River

NEW JERSEY AND NEW YORK

NEW YORK–NEW JERSEY TRAIL CONFERENCE
156 Ramapo Valley Road (Route 202)

Mahwah, NJ 07430-1199
(201) 512-9348
www.nynjtc.org
Delaware River to Connecticut–New York
border

CONNECTICUT AND MASSACHUSETTS

AMC Connecticut Chapter
964 South Main Street
Great Barrington, MA 01230
(413) 528-6333
www.ct–amc.org
Connecticut–New York border to Sages
Ravine

AMC–BERKSHIRE CHAPTER
964 South Main Street
Great Barrington, MA 01230
(413) 528-6333
www.amcberkshire.org
Sages Ravine to Vermont–Massachusetts
border

VERMONT, NEW HAMPSHIRE, AND MAINE

GREEN MOUNTAIN CLUB
4711 Waterbury–Stowe Road
Waterbury Center, VT 05677
(802) 244-7037
www.greenmountainclub.org
Vermont–Massachusetts border to VT 12

DARTMOUTH OUTING CLUB
P. O. Box 9
Hanover, NH 03755
(603) 646-2428
www.dartmouth.edu/~doc
VT 12 to Kinsman Notch, NH

APPALACHIAN MOUNTAIN CLUB
PINKHAM NOTCH CAMP
P. O. Box 298
Gorham, NH 03581-0298
(603) 466-2721
www.outdoors.org
Kinsman Notch, NH, to Grafton Notch, ME

TRAIL MAINTENANCE CLUBS *(continued)*

MAINE APPALACHIAN TRAIL CLUB
P. O. Box 283
Augusta, ME 04332-0283
www.matc.org
Grafton Notch to Katahdin, ME

OF RELATED INTEREST

APPALACHIAN LONG DISTANCE HIKERS
ASSOCIATION (ALDHA)
10 Benning Street, PMB 224
West Lebanon, NH 03784
www.aldha.org
*Organizes work trips on the A.T. and an
annual "Gathering" featuring workshops
and presentations.*

KEYSTONE TRAILS ASSOCIATION
P. O. Box 129
Confluence, PA 15424
www.kta–hike.org
*KTA is the umbrella organization for clubs
throughout Pennsylvania, some of which
maintain the A.T.*

A.T. CLUB OF FLORIDA
c/o Grace Tyner
1310 Quail Drive
Sarasota, FL 34231
(941) 921-1467
gatyner@ix.netcom.com
ATC Supporting Organization

A.T. CLUB OF ALABAMA
P. O. Box 381842
Birmingham, AL 35238
www.sport.al.com/sport/atca

LOWER APPALACHIAN TRAIL ASSOCIATION
507 Broadway
Sylacauga, AL 35150

ILLINOIS A.T. CLUB
c/o Norbert Simon
1508 Hinman Avenue, Apt. 4-B
Evanston, IL 60201
(847) 869-9818
nasimon4@attbi.com

INTERNATIONAL APPALACHIAN TRAIL
27 Flying Point Road
Freeport, ME 04032
(207) 865-6233
www.internationalat.org

A.T. HOME PAGE
www.fred.net/kathy/at.html

TRAILPLACE
www.trailplace.com

WHITEBLAZE.NET
www.whiteblaze.net

INDEX

ABOUT THE
AUTHORS

Frank and Victoria Logue hiked the entire Appalachian Trail in 1988. They have returned again and again to hike its many sections on day and overnight hikes. Frank served on the Appalachian Trail Conservancy Board of Managers. The Logues live in Georgia where Frank works as an Episcopal priest while Victoria writes. They both enjoy sharing their love of nature with their daughter, Griffin.

Leonard M. Adkins has been intimately involved with the Appalachian Trail for more than two decades. He has hiked its full length four times, and lacks just a few hundred miles to complete it for a fifth. He was a ridgerunner for the Appalachian Trail Conservancy and is presently an A.T. Natural Heritage Site Monitor, aiding the conservancy and the National Park Service in overseeing the welfare of rare and endangered plants. In addition, he currently serves on the Board of Directors of the Roanoke Appalachian Trail Club and maintains a section of the A.T. near McAfee Knob. Among the other long-distance trails Leonard has completed are the Continental Divide Trail from Canada to Mexico, Pacific Northwest Trail from Glacier National Park to the Pacific Ocean, and the Pyrenees High Route along the border of France and Spain. In all, he has walked more than 17,000 miles exploring the backcountry areas of the United States, Canada, Europe, and the Caribbean. Leonard is the author of more than ten books on travel and the outdoors. His *Wildflowers of the Appalachian Trail* was presented the National Outdoor Book Award, while *The Appalachian Trail: A Visitor's Companion*, received the Lowell Thomas Travel Journalism Award. He also writes the hiking columns for *The Roanoker* and *Blue Ridge Outdoors* magazines. Along with this thru-hiking wife, Laurie, and thru-hiking dog, MacAfee of Knob, he lives in the Catawba Valley of Virginia, just a few miles from the A.T.